CW00750558

The Fibromyalgia Mastery Bible: Your Blueprint For Complete Fibromyalgia Management

Dr. Ankita Kashyap and Prof. Krishna N. Sharma

Published by Virtued Press, 2023.

While every precaution has been taken in the preparation of this book, the publisher assumes no responsibility for errors or omissions, or for damages resulting from the use of the information contained herein.

THE FIBROMYALGIA MASTERY BIBLE: YOUR BLUEPRINT FOR COMPLETE FIBROMYALGIA MANAGEMENT

First edition. November 20, 2023.

Copyright © 2023 Dr. Ankita Kashyap and Prof. Krishna N. Sharma.

ISBN: 979-8223175766

Written by Dr. Ankita Kashyap and Prof. Krishna N. Sharma.

Table of Contents

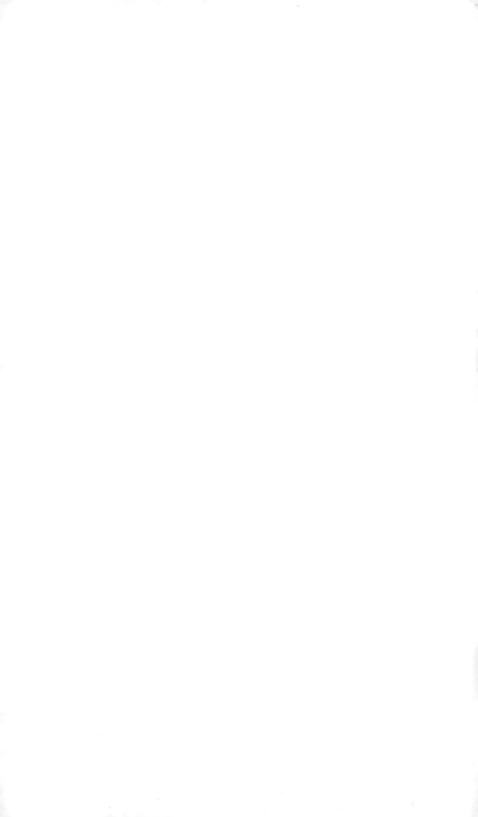

DISCLAIMER

The information provided in this book is intended for general informational purposes only. The content is not meant to substitute professional medical advice, diagnosis, or treatment. Always consult with a qualified healthcare provider before making any changes to your diabetes management plan or healthcare regimen.

While every effort has been made to ensure the accuracy and completeness of the information presented, the author and publisher do not assume any responsibility for errors, omissions, or potential misinterpretations of the content. Individual responses to diabetes management strategies may vary, and what works for one person might not be suitable for another.

The book does not endorse any specific medical treatments, products, or services. Readers are encouraged to seek guidance from their healthcare providers to determine the most appropriate approaches for their unique medical conditions and needs.

Any external links or resources provided in the book are for convenience and informational purposes only. The author and publisher do not have control over the content or availability of these external sources and do not endorse or guarantee the accuracy of such information.

Readers are advised to exercise caution and use their judgment when applying the information provided in this book to their own situations. The author and publisher disclaim any liability for any direct, indirect, consequential, or other damages arising from the use of this book and its content.

By reading and using this book, readers acknowledge and accept the limitations and inherent risks associated with implementing the strategies, recommendations, and information contained herein. It is always recommended to consult a qualified healthcare professional for personalized medical advice and care.

Introduction

I can't help but be amazed at the world of possibilities that lie ahead as I sit here with a pen in hand and a flutter of joy in my heart. I'm going to take you on a voyage today, dear reader, a big expedition into the depths of empowerment, insight, and wisdom. Together, we will tackle the wide territory of fibromyalgia, solve its riddles, and find the secrets to understanding this sometimes mysterious condition.

Greetings from The Fibromyalgia Mastery Bible: Your Complete Guide to Fibromyalgia Management, my dear friends. I offer this beautiful quilt of wisdom, understanding, and direction as a sincere gift to everyone who has been ensnared by the confusing conditions that bind them. I knew I had found my vocation and calling as soon as I laid eyes on the complex network of fibromyalgia.

In the medical field, where technical terms and intricacy are frequently king, my goal is to simplify the complexities of fibromyalgia while incorporating a whimsical and endearing touch. I will use soft words, a slow pace, and a dash of fairy dust to add levity to this heavy subject matter, much like a good painter employs subtle brushstrokes to bring life to their canvases.

Envision, if you will, strolling through the knowledge meadows, with every step carrying the aroma of opportunity. The grass feels smooth underfoot, like a plush carpet brushing against your feet. The sun dances across your skin, infusing your entire soul with warmth and the certainty that the answers you seek are just a short distance away. The soft air whispers hope.

I am going to be your guide in this precious place where holistic health and medicine meet. I have assembled an impressive team of professionals from a range of health and wellness domains, using my years of medical experience and my enthusiasm for all-encompassing healthcare. We will work together to create a tapestry of understanding that will provide you a variety of viewpoints, each of which will be finely woven into the fabric of your own experience.

I swear to hold your hand with unfailing understanding and compassion as we delve further into this engrossing storey. Every page has been thoughtfully created by me with the goal of providing ample value along with deep knowledge. You see, dear reader, our goal is to provide you with practical solutions that will enable you to navigate the complex ins and outs of fibromyalgia like a compass. It is not enough for us to merely grasp the illness.

Like a complicated tapestry, fibromyalgia manifests itself as a kaleidoscope of symptoms that are specific to each person and resemble a thumbprint of agony. With this deep comprehension in mind, let me present the idea of adaptable strategies and self-help methods. You will discover a haven of opportunities within the pages of this book, where you can create a wellness road map that melds perfectly with the details of your personal trip.

To my dear reader, I beg you to open your mind and let us delve into the wide world of medical and complementary therapies for fibromyalgia. Together, we will explore topics such as dietary and lifestyle planning, counselling, psychology, alternative forms of self-care, complementary therapies, and coping mechanisms.

I extend an invitation to you to go on a life-changing journey through the pages of this book, one that will not only teach you new things but also help you rediscover your inner resilience and strength. Though the road ahead may seem difficult, I can promise you that the benefits will be incalculable. I hope you feel lighter, more liberated, and more in control than ever as we peel back the layers of misconception around fibromyalgia and reveal its secrets.

Now, grab my hand, my reader, and let's explore this amazing knowledge tapestry. Allow the words on these pages to tell a tale of recovery, optimism, and overcoming hardship. By working together, we can overcome the effects of fibromyalgia and take control of our own fate. Are you set to go? Then let's start this amazing adventure together.

Chapter 1: Understanding Fibromyalgia

The Science Behind Fibromyalgia

Millions of people worldwide are afflicted with the complicated fibromyalgia ailment. My mission as a physician and health and wellness coach is to provide you a thorough grasp of the science underlying fibromyalgia so you can take charge of your health and successfully manage your symptoms.

We must first examine the neurological and physiological components of fibromyalgia in order to fully appreciate its complexity. New discoveries in science have illuminated the fundamental processes that lead to the onset and persistence of fibromyalgia symptoms.

Central sensitization is one of these mechanisms. The central nervous system hypersensitivity that characterises fibromyalgia patients causes an exaggerated pain response to stimuli that are not normally thought to be uncomfortable. It is believed that an imbalance in neurotransmitters, which are chemical messengers that help nerve cells communicate with one another, is the source of this hypersensitivity.

The body's regulation of pain perception and transmission is greatly influenced by neurotransmitters. Studies have indicated that fibromyalgia patients have changed levels of serotonin, dopamine, and norepinephrine, among other neurotransmitters. These neurotransmitters play a role in mood, pain sensitivity, and sleep regulation. Patients with fibromyalgia may have widespread pain and other symptoms due to imbalances in these neurotransmitters.

One neurotransmitter that controls mood, hunger, sleep, and pain is serotonin. Studies have indicated that serotonin levels may be lowered in fibromyalgia patients, which may account for symptoms including anxiety, melancholy, exhaustion, and reduced pain threshold. We can investigate methods to raise serotonin levels and alleviate symptoms by comprehending the function of serotonin in fibromyalgia.

Dopamine, a neurotransmitter linked to motivation, reward, and pleasure, is also implicated in fibromyalgia. Research has indicated that alterations in dopamine levels may be present in fibromyalgia patients, potentially exacerbating symptoms such as fatigue, cognitive impairments, and reduced desire. We can take action to alleviate these symptoms and improve general wellbeing by treating dopamine abnormalities.

Furthermore, fibromyalgia has been linked to norepinephrine, a neurotransmitter that controls the body's stress response. Studies have indicated that norepinephrine dysregulation in fibromyalgia patients may be responsible for their elevated stress response and heightened sensitivity to pain. Norepinephrine abnormalities may be treated in order to potentially lessen discomfort and enhance the body's capacity to handle stress.

Knowing how neurotransmitters function in fibromyalgia gives us a solid basis for creating symptom management plans. Making changes to one's lifestyle is one such tactic that can assist control neurotransmitter levels and enhance general wellbeing. Frequent exercise, for instance, has been demonstrated to raise dopamine and serotonin levels, which improve mood and pain tolerance. Including low-impact workouts, yoga, tai chi, or other similar activities can help manage the symptoms of fibromyalgia.

One important feature of fibromyalgia is faulty pain processing, in addition to neurotransmitter abnormalities. Studies have revealed that people with fibromyalgia have different brain circuits for processing pain, which makes them more sensitive to pain. Patients with fibromyalgia may suffer broad pain as a result of this aberrant pain processing, which can prolong the pain cycle.

Knowing the neurological component of fibromyalgia enables us to investigate different self-care practises and coping mechanisms that may be useful in managing symptoms. For instance, cognitive-behavioral therapy (CBT) is a successful therapeutic strategy that can assist people in changing the way they think and feel about pain, lowering their levels of anxiety and depression, and improving their general ability to manage pain. Through cognitive behavioural therapy (CBT) and other psychological approaches, we can address the neurological component of fibromyalgia and enable people to actively manage their symptoms.

Furthermore, complementary and alternative therapies like biofeedback, mindfulness meditation, and acupuncture have demonstrated promise in the management of fibromyalgia symptoms. These methods function by influencing how the brain reacts to pain and encouraging calmness and a reduction in tension. We may enhance our well-being and quality of life by adding these self-help methods to our toolset for managing fibromyalgia.

We may learn a great deal about the neurological and physiological components of fibromyalgia from scientific study. Through an appreciation of the functions of neurotransmitters, central sensitization, and aberrant pain processing, we can create a customised strategy for the treatment of fibromyalgia symptoms. Self-care practises, coping mechanisms, and lifestyle adjustments can help us take back control of our health and wellbeing.

We will examine how nutrition and diet affect fibromyalgia in the upcoming chapter and go over methods for maximising our dietary intake to help manage fibromyalgia. Come along as we explore the realm of nutrition and learn about the foods that can nourish our bodies and reduce discomfort. We may set out on a journey together to live a life that is healthier and more lively.

Recognizing the Symptoms

Widespread pain is one of the main signs and symptoms of fibromyalgia. Many people describe this pain as a deep, painful sensation that spreads to many parts of the body. Tenderness in certain trigger points, such as the neck, shoulders, chest, hips, and knees, may also accompany it. This all-over discomfort, which can be intermittent or continuous, can seriously lower your quality of life and make even the most basic chores difficult.

Another typical symptom that people with fibromyalgia often encounter is fatigue. It is an intense feeling of physical and mental tiredness that lasts long after resting, not merely a tired feeling after a hard day. It can be extremely difficult to perform daily tasks, job, or maintain social interactions while fatigued. It is critical to realise that this weariness is a physiological symptom of the illness rather than the result of laziness or lack of ambition.

People with fibromyalgia also frequently experience sleep difficulties. Many people have trouble falling asleep, remaining asleep, or getting a good night's sleep. People may experience restless sleep as a result, waking up feeling drained and underslept. Sleep problems can have a detrimental effect on mood, cognition, and general wellbeing in addition to exacerbating fatigue.

One of the less well-known signs of fibromyalgia is cognitive impairments, or "fibro fog," which can significantly affect day-to-day functioning. Many people who have fibromyalgia report having memory, focus, and mental clarity issues. Simple tasks could become difficult, and people can find it difficult to remember knowledge or follow conversations. This cognitive impairment can cause worry, dissatisfaction, and problems both personally and professionally.

Apart from the widely known symptoms, fibromyalgia can also cause a wide range of additional symptoms. Even though these symptoms are less frequently acknowledged, they can nevertheless have a big impact on a person's day-to-day activities. For instance, it's common to hear of people developing increased sensitivity to touch, light, sound, and temperature. This increased sensitivity may cause discomfort and necessitate avoiding particular situations or stimuli.

Furthermore, gastrointestinal problems including irritable bowel syndrome are common in people with fibromyalgia (IBS). Abdominal pain, bloating, diarrhoea, or constipation are possible presentations of this. The unpredictability of these digestive problems can lead to extra stress and discomfort, which worsens general health.

Mood disorders, including anxiety and sadness, are very commonly seen in fibromyalgia sufferers. Stress levels might rise and emotions of melancholy and pessimism can result from dealing with chronic pain, exhaustion, and other symptoms. In order to support complete well-being, it is imperative to address these emotional disorders in addition to the physical symptoms.

Lastly, it's critical to understand that fibromyalgia can have varying effects on various people. Even though these are some of the most often reported symptoms, each individual may experience symptoms that differ in intensity and appearance. Since every person's experience with fibromyalgia is different, it is essential to monitor and treat each patient as an individual.

Effective fibromyalgia management begins with an understanding of these symptoms. You can create coping mechanisms and techniques to reduce symptoms by realising the problems that chronic pain, exhaustion, sleep disturbances, cognitive issues, and other symptoms present.

We will examine each symptom in more detail in the upcoming chapters, looking at potential causes, underlying mechanisms, and management approaches. Together, we will develop a thorough plan for managing your fibromyalgia completely, giving you the ability to take back control of your life and seek relief from the crippling symptoms of this illness.

Diagnosing Fibromyalgia

Fibromyalgia diagnosis can be difficult to make. It necessitates a meticulous assessment of the patient as well as a comprehensive comprehension of the symptoms. To achieve precise diagnoses, our clinic combines more recent, comprehensive recommendations with more established techniques like the tender point examination.

The gold standard for fibromyalgia diagnosis has historically been the tender point examination. This diagnostic method, created by the American College of Rheumatology, uses pressure to target particular body sites to identify any sore or irritated areas. There are sore points in many different places, such as the knees, hips, shoulders, and neck.

I carefully palpate each of these places during the tender point examination in order to gauge the patient's pain threshold. I use my fingertips to apply steady pressure, building it up gradually until the patient complains of pain. This enables me to gauge how severe their symptoms are and how high they can tolerate pain.

But in recent years, there has been more scrutiny of the tender point test. According to some experts, it might not fully capture the intricacy of fibromyalgia. They contend that it may ignore other significant symptoms that patients have in favour of an overemphasis on pain.

More recent diagnostic criteria have been created in response to these worries. The widespread pain index (WPI) and symptom severity scale (SSS) is one such recommendation that combines a greater variety of symptoms and their intensity to offer a more precise diagnosis of fibromyalgia. This method considers not only pain but also weariness, insomnia, problems with cognition, and other related symptoms.

In my opinion as a holistic healthcare professional, these more recent diagnostic guidelines provide a more thorough grasp of the illness. A patient's quality of life may be greatly impacted by a variety of physical and psychological symptoms that are included in fibromyalgia, which goes beyond pain. By taking into account every facet of the illness, we are able to offer more individualised and efficient treatment programmes.

Still, there are difficulties and disagreements with the fibromyalgia diagnosis. One problem is that there are no objective tests or particular biomarkers to identify the illness. In contrast to other medical diseases, fibromyalgia cannot be identified by blood work or imaging studies. This may lead to suspicion from some in the medical community and make it challenging for medical practitioners to reach a firm diagnosis.

Moreover, the diagnostic process may be complicated by the similarities between fibromyalgia and other illnesses such rheumatoid arthritis and chronic fatigue syndrome. It necessitates a thorough assessment of the patient's medical background, a physical examination, and the rule out of other possible reasons for their symptoms.

The subjective nature of pain and other symptoms that fibromyalgia sufferers perceive presents another difficulty. The pain associated with fibromyalgia is frequently imperceptible to others, in contrast to apparent injuries or shattered bones. This might result in a lack of empathy and understanding from the medical community as well as from society at large.

Despite these difficulties, fibromyalgia diagnosis is essential for efficient care and management. For those who have frequently suffered for years without receiving assistance, it offers validation. It also helps medical practitioners create individualised treatment programmes that cater to the particular requirements of every patient.

In order to guarantee an accurate diagnosis, I place a strong emphasis on the value of a thorough history taking and physical examination in my practise. In order to find any patterns or triggers that might be causing my patients' illness, I pay close attention to their symptoms and thoroughly examine their medical histories. Having a comprehensive grasp of the situation allows us to better manage fibromyalgia overall and customise our treatment plans.

Additionally, I think it's important to validate the experiences of my patients. Fibromyalgia is a complicated and frequently misdiagnosed illness. I provide my patients the tools they need to take charge of their health and speak up for themselves by realising the impact it has on their life.

In summary, a combination of more recent, thorough guidelines and more conventional diagnostic techniques, such the tender point examination, are used to diagnose fibromyalgia. Although the tender point examination has been the norm for a long time, more recent standards offer a more comprehensive assessment of the situation. There are difficulties and disagreements related to diagnosing fibromyalgia, such as the absence of certain biomarkers and the subjective character of symptoms. On the other hand, a precise diagnosis is essential for validating the condition and permitting efficient management and therapy. By means of a thorough evaluation and customised methodology, medical practitioners can enable their patients to assume responsibility for their fibromyalgia path.

Demographics and Prevalence

Worldwide, people with fibromyalgia, a chronic pain illness, come from a variety of demographic backgrounds. It is frequently misunderstood to be a disorder that mostly affects women or older persons. On the other hand, current investigations and studies have demonstrated that fibromyalgia can impact anyone of any age, gender, or ethnicity.

First, let's look at how common fibromyalgia is among various age groups. Even while the illness can strike anyone at any age, people between the ages of 20 and 55 are the ones who are typically diagnosed with it. People typically juggle a lot of responsibilities at this period of life, from work to family and everything in between. This busy stage of life may lead to elevated stress levels and weakened immune systems, which in turn may contribute to the high prevalence of fibromyalgia in this age range.

Let's talk about how gender impacts fibromyalgia. It is true that women are disproportionately affected by this ailment. In fact, it's thought that women may account for up to 90% of fibromyalgia diagnoses. Although the exact causes of this gender gap are still being investigated, it is thought that hormonal variables, genetic predispositions, and variations in how men and women perceive pain all be important contributors. While men can also experience fibromyalgia, these cases are much less common.

While it would seem that the prevalence of fibromyalgia is the same across all ethnic groups, research indicates otherwise. Research has indicated that fibromyalgia is more common in several ethnic groups, especially with people who identify as Caucasian. There are a number of potential causes for this variation in prevalence, including genetic variants, disparities in socioeconomic level, and variations in healthcare availability. To pinpoint the precise causes of this disparity, more research is necessary.

14

Let's now investigate how social and cultural aspects affect how fibromyalgia is perceived and treated. Similar to numerous other chronic illnesses, fibromyalgia is impacted by cultural attitudes and beliefs. For instance, people with fibromyalgia may feel alone or ashamed of their illness because chronic pain is stigmatised in some cultures. This may make it more difficult for them to get the support and care they need.

Furthermore, the way fibromyalgia symptoms are expressed and described is also influenced by cultural influences. Accurately diagnosing and treating fibromyalgia across cultural boundaries can be difficult for healthcare practitioners due to differences in descriptions and interpretations of pain. Furthermore, how people deal with chronic pain may also be influenced by cultural norms and expectations, which can affect how well management techniques work.

Furthermore, the way fibromyalgia is managed can be significantly impacted by societal factors like socioeconomic status and access to healthcare. It may be more difficult for people from lower socioeconomic backgrounds to get proper medical treatment, including access to experts and prescription drugs. Financial limitations may also prevent them from accessing self-help methods or alternative therapies that might be used in addition to conventional medical care.

In conclusion, although there are differences in prevalence across these groups, fibromyalgia affects people of all ages, genders, and ethnicities. The understanding, diagnosis, and treatment of fibromyalgia are all influenced by cultural and societal aspects, which are important in how the disorder is perceived and managed. Healthcare practitioners can customise their approach to managing fibromyalgia and ensure that individuals receive the necessary support and resources by taking these demographics and cultural factors into account.

Chapter 2: Medical Management of Fibromyalgia

Medications for Fibromyalgia

The most common and incapacitating fibromyalgia symptom is pain. It has an impact on every element of a person's life, making it challenging to go about everyday tasks and lead a fulfilling existence. As a physician with a focus on holistic medicine and wellness, my goal is to assist patients in properly managing their pain and regaining control over their lives.

Using painkillers is one of the first lines of treatment for fibromyalgia pain. NSAIDs, or nonsteroidal anti-inflammatory medicines, are frequently recommended to treat pain and inflammation. Examples of NSAIDs include ibuprofen and naproxen. These drugs function by preventing the body from producing specific molecules that cause pain and inflammation. Although NSAIDs have been shown to be helpful in certain situations, they are not usually enough to treat the persistent pain that comes with fibromyalgia.

Opioids are a different family of painkillers that are frequently used to treat fibromyalgia pain. Opioids lessen the experience of pain by attaching to opioid receptors in the brain and spinal cord. Opioids have a number of hazards and adverse effects, including the possibility of addiction and dependency, even if they can be quite effective in relieving pain. As a result, opioids are typically saved for extremely severe fibromyalgia pain that does not improve with other forms of therapy.

For fibromyalgia, antidepressant drugs are frequently administered in addition to pain medicines. Some people might find this surprising because fibromyalgia is not usually categorised as a mental illness. Nonetheless, studies have demonstrated that antidepressants can help fibromyalgia sufferers feel better overall and with less discomfort.

Selective serotonin reuptake inhibitors are one class of antidepressants that is frequently prescribed for fibromyalgia (SSRIs). Serotonin helps control mood and lessens perception of pain, and

SSRIs function by raising serotonin levels in the brain. Examples of SSRIs that are frequently administered for fibromyalgia are escitalopram, sertraline, and fluoxetine.

Tricyclic antidepressants are another type of antidepressants that are frequently recommended for fibromyalgia (TCAs). TCAs relieve pain by raising the amounts of substances in the brain that are involved in it, like norepinephrine and serotonin. Two TCAs that are frequently used for fibromyalgia are amitriptyline and nortriptyline.

Antidepressants not only relieve pain but also aid with sleep quality and weariness, two frequent fibromyalgia symptoms. Antidepressants may not have their full effects for several weeks, so it's vital to be patient and give them time to do their job.

Anticonvulsant drugs, which were first created to treat epilepsy, have demonstrated potential in the treatment of fibromyalgia pain. By calming down the brain's overactive nerves, these drugs help lessen the perception of pain. For fibromyalgia, gabapentin and pregabalin are the anticonvulsants that are most frequently administered.

Anticonvulsants not only aid with pain relief but also with sleep, fatigue reduction, and the feelings of anxiety and depression, which are frequently linked to fibromyalgia.

It's important to remember that not every patient should take every drug. The symptoms of the patient, their medical history, and the existence of any additional medical disorders all play a role in the pharmaceutical selection process. Before beginning any new treatment, it is important to thoroughly assess the risks and side effects that are specific to each prescription.

For a thorough and all-encompassing treatment strategy, drugs should be used in conjunction with other non-pharmacological treatments, even though they can play a significant role in the management of fibromyalgia. Healthy nutrition, stress reduction, and regular exercise are just a few examples of lifestyle changes that can greatly lessen the symptoms of fibromyalgia and lessen the need for medication.

In summary, drugs are essential for controlling fibromyalgia pain and related symptoms. Antidepressants, anticonvulsants, and painkillers are frequently administered to patients in an effort to alleviate their symptoms and enhance their general health. To choose the right drug and dosage for each patient, it's crucial to collaborate closely with a healthcare provider. Furthermore, for a complete and all-encompassing management strategy, medicine should always be used in conjunction with other non-pharmacological approaches. People with fibromyalgia can recover control over their life and experience symptom alleviation with the correct care and assistance.

Physical Therapies and Rehabilitation

When done properly and in moderation, exercise can be a very effective technique for controlling the symptoms of fibromyalgia. For this reason, many people who suffer from fibromyalgia avoid physical exercise for fear of making their pain or exhaustion worse. Nonetheless, numerous studies have consistently demonstrated that engaging in regular exercise can result in notable enhancements in pain perception, physical capabilities, and general quality of life.

According to a study that was published in the Journal of Rheumatology, fibromyalgia sufferers who engaged in a 12-week fitness regimen had improvements in their levels of exhaustion and despair as well as a decrease in the intensity of their pain. It is crucial to remember that physical activity should be customised to meet the unique demands and capabilities of each person. This is where a physiotherapist's or exercise specialist's experience is useful.

Physical therapy, or physiotherapy, can play a crucial role in a person's fibromyalgia treatment strategy. Physiotherapists are qualified to evaluate abnormal movement patterns, muscle weakness, and biomechanical abnormalities in the body. Physiotherapy can assist in restoring joint mobility, lowering muscular tension, and improving posture by addressing these underlying problems.

Manual therapy is a typical technique used in physiotherapy for fibromyalgia. Using a hands-on approach, the therapist manipulates soft tissues, mobilises joints, and relieves pain using a variety of manual treatments. Improved blood flow, relaxation, and a reduction in painful areas are all possible with manual treatment.

Exercise therapy is an additional component of physiotherapy for fibromyalgia. A physiotherapist can create a personalised workout plan that takes into consideration the goals, symptoms, and existing fitness level of the patient. A mix of cardiovascular, strengthening, and stretching activities may be included of the programme. The idea is to minimise the risk of overdoing it or getting hurt while progressively increasing physical activity and endurance.

Occupational therapy enhances physical treatment by concentrating on enhancing a person's capacity to carry out daily tasks. Occupational therapists collaborate with patients to pinpoint any obstacles or constraints they might be experiencing and devise plans of action to surmount them. This could entail making adjustments to the living space, offering assistive technology, or imparting energy-saving knowledge.

Individuals with fibromyalgia who took part in an occupational therapy programme demonstrated significant improvements in pain, exhaustion, and functioning, according to a study published in the American Journal of Occupational Therapy. Along with useful tips for handling everyday chores, the seminar covered energy saving, stress management, and activity pacing.

People with fibromyalgia may get relief from alternative physical therapies and rehabilitation methods in addition to exercise, physiotherapy, and occupational therapy. These could consist of chiropractic adjustments, hydrotherapy, acupuncture, and massage therapy. Many people claim to receive relief and relaxation from these techniques, while individual results may vary in their usefulness.

For example, massage therapy has been shown to help people with fibromyalgia feel better overall, sleep better, and lessen discomfort. Significant pain intensity reductions and increases in sleep quality can result from massage therapy, according to a meta-analysis published in the Journal of Clinical Rheumatology.

For those suffering from fibromyalgia, hydrotherapy—which is the use of water for therapeutic purposes—can be helpful. Water's buoyancy makes it possible for mild movements and stretching exercises while also easing the strain on joints and muscles. According to a study that was published in the European Journal of Physical and

Rehabilitation Medicine, fibromyalgia patients' pain, weariness, and general functioning all improved with hydrotherapy.

In order to reestablish the flow of energy in the body, tiny needles are inserted into certain body sites during acupuncture, a type of traditional Chinese medicine. According to some study, acupuncture may help fibromyalgia sufferers sleep better and feel less pain. To properly comprehend its efficacy, further excellent research is necessary.

People with fibromyalgia may also benefit from chiropractic care, which focuses on the diagnosis and treatment of mechanical abnormalities of the musculoskeletal system. Spinal manipulations are among the manual treatments used by chiropractors to correct the spine's and joints' alignment and function. Although there is no evidence on chiropractic care specifically for fibromyalgia, several patients claim that these treatments have improved their mobility and provided pain relief.

It is significant to remember that individual differences may exist in the efficacy of these physical therapy and rehabilitation methods. Finding the ideal mix of therapies that yields the greatest benefit may need some trial and error as what works for one person may not necessarily work for another. Working with licenced medical specialists who are skilled in treating fibromyalgia and can customise treatment regimens to meet each patient's needs is also very important.

To sum up, physical therapy and rehabilitation have shown to be effective strategies for managing fibromyalgia. Mobility, discomfort, and general quality of life can all be enhanced with the use of exercise, physiotherapy, and occupational therapy. Furthermore, some people may benefit further from additional physical therapies such massage therapy, hydrotherapy, acupuncture, and chiropractic care. People with fibromyalgia can improve their sense of well-being and have more control over their symptoms by combining various therapy modalities. As a holistic medical professional, I'm dedicated to giving my patients all-encompassing care that takes into account not just the physical aspects of their illness but also their mental and emotional wellness. By working together, we can develop a customised treatment plan that gives people the tools they need to take control of their fibromyalgia journey and lead happy, full lives.

Complementary and Alternative Medicine

I really think that treating fibromyalgia holistically is the best course of action. I have personally witnessed the advantages of integrating complementary and alternative medicine (CAM) into an all-encompassing treatment plan, even if mainstream medicine undoubtedly has its advantages. In addition to treating the physical side of fibromyalgia, complementary and alternative medicine (CAM) considers the patient's emotional, mental, and spiritual health.

Acupuncture is one of the CAM therapies for fibromyalgia that is most well-known and researched. In this traditional Chinese medicine, tiny needles are inserted into predetermined bodily locations. Traditional Chinese medicine holds that the body's life force, or qi, is carried by passageways called meridians that connect these locations. Acupuncture attempts to balance the body and restore qi flow by activating these sites.

Numerous studies have demonstrated the potential benefit of acupuncture in treating fibromyalgia. Researchers showed that acupuncture was much more effective than sham acupuncture in lowering pain and enhancing quality of life in individuals with fibromyalgia. The results of the trial were reported in the Journal of Rehabilitation Medicine. A different study on fibromyalgia patients revealed that acupuncture reduced pain intensity, exhaustion, and sleep disturbances. This study was also published in the Journal of Alternative and Complementary Medicine.

Traditional medical systems have traditionally employed herbal medicines in addition to acupuncture to treat chronic pain and inflammation. Turmeric is one herb whose potential benefits in managing fibromyalgia have come to light. Curcumin, a substance present in turmeric, has been shown to have analgesic and anti-inflammatory effects. A randomised controlled experiment that was published in the Journal of Clinical Psychopharmacology revealed that fibromyalgia patients' quality of life was greatly enhanced and pain was dramatically reduced when they took curcumin supplements.

Herbal medicines such as St. John's wort, ginger, and lavender have also demonstrated potential in the management of fibromyalgia symptoms. One major comorbidity of fibromyalgia is depression, which is sometimes treated with St. John's wort. On the other hand, ginger is a great option for people who are in pain or have inflammation because it has been shown to have anti-inflammatory and analgesic qualities. Due to its relaxing and soothing qualities, lavender is well-known for helping fibromyalgia sufferers relax and get better sleep.

Research has demonstrated the efficacy of mind-body therapies, including yoga and mindfulness-based stress reduction (MBSR), in mitigating pain and enhancing overall quality of life among individuals suffering from fibromyalgia. The Jon Kabat-Zinn-created MBSR method combines body awareness practises, moderate yoga, and mindfulness meditation. Studies have indicated that taking part in MBSR programmes can result in notable enhancements in pain, exhaustion, and general quality of life for individuals with fibromyalgia.

In a similar vein, yoga has been demonstrated to be helpful for those with fibromyalgia. Yoga therapies significantly reduced pain and exhaustion, improved sleep quality, and improved physical performance in fibromyalgia patients, according to a comprehensive review and meta-analysis published in the journal Pain Medicine.

It is crucial to treat the person's entire lifestyle and well-being in addition to these particular complementary and alternative therapies. This entails adjusting one's lifestyle as needed, such as increasing exercise on a regular basis, maintaining proper sleep hygiene, and controlling stress. The psychological and emotional difficulties of having fibromyalgia can be more effectively managed by people with the aid of counselling and psychology-related strategies.

I collaborate closely with a group of professionals from different health and wellness domains in my practise to offer a thorough approach to managing fibromyalgia. To give each of our patients a customised treatment plan that meets their specific needs, we integrate complementary and alternative medicine with conventional therapy.

To sum up, complementary and alternative medicine provides useful choices for the treatment of fibromyalgia. These therapies, which range from mind-body therapy to herbal remedies and acupuncture, can help relieve pain, lower inflammation, promote better sleep, and improve general wellbeing. People can find relief and recover control of their life by managing their fibromyalgia holistically, including complementary and alternative medicine (CAM) therapies.

Interventional Treatments

Trigger point injections are one interventional therapy that has demonstrated promise in the management of fibromyalgia. For those with fibromyalgia, trigger points—hypersensitive spots in the muscles—can be a major source of discomfort. These injections entail injecting a combination of anaesthetic and anti-inflammatory medicine into these trigger sites using a tiny needle. Reducing muscle tension and easing discomfort in the afflicted areas is the goal.

Injections into trigger points have the potential to quickly and locally reduce pain. The anti-inflammatory drug aids in reducing inflammation and promoting healing while the anaesthetic numbs the affected area. It's crucial to understand that trigger point injections are a technique for managing fibromyalgia symptoms rather than a treatment for the condition. Each person may respond differently to these injections, and some may need more than one to experience long-lasting pain relief.

Injections using trigger points may be useful for some people, but not everyone may benefit from them. Before recommending this surgery, it is imperative to evaluate the medical history, anatomic concerns, and general state of health of each patient. Furthermore, since each patient has unique triggers and pain spots, it is imperative to customise the treatment approach.

Neural blocks are an additional interventional therapy for fibromyalgia that is worth investigating. In order to block pain signals, local anaesthetic medicine is injected close to particular nerves in a procedure known as a nerve block. Neural blocks for fibromyalgia may target the neurons responsible for transmitting pain signals from trigger sites or tender points.

The main objective of nerve blocks is to stop pain impulses and deliver relief. Patients may lessen the frequency and intensity of their pain by inhibiting the nerve signals that cause pain. It's crucial to

27

remember that nerve blocks are a temporary fix and may need to be repeated in order to keep the pain at bay.

Nerve blocks must to be performed carefully and under a qualified healthcare provider's supervision. Although they may be advantageous for certain people, they come with a risk profile and possible adverse consequences. Before beginning any treatment, it is crucial to carefully assess each patient's eligibility for it and go over the possible advantages, hazards, and other possibilities.

Spinal cord stimulation is a possible interventional treatment for fibromyalgia in certain situations where other treatments have not worked. A tiny gadget, like a pacemaker, is inserted beneath the lower back's skin to stimulate the spinal cord. By producing electrical impulses that obstruct pain signals as they go via the spinal cord, the gadget lessens the sensation of pain.

In contrast to trigger point injections and nerve blocks, spinal cord stimulation is a more intrusive operation. It necessitates the device's surgical implantation, usually carried out under local anaesthetic. Electrodes are positioned in close proximity to the spinal cord and linked to a patient-controlled pulse generator during the process. It is possible to modify the electrical impulses' frequency and strength to meet the needs of each individual.

Even though spinal cord stimulation has demonstrated promise in the management of chronic pain, including fibromyalgia, it is crucial to evaluate and carefully examine spinal cord stimulation as a treatment option before pursuing it. Usually saved as a last resort, this operation is performed on people whose severe pain has not improved despite trying several therapies.

It is critical to take into account the patient's overall health, medical history, pain profile, and treatment goals prior to proposing any interventional treatment. To ascertain the appropriateness of these treatments, their possible advantages, and the associated dangers, a complete examination that includes a conversation with the patient is necessary.

Interventional therapies must always be used sparingly and in conjunction with a thorough management strategy for fibromyalgia. They are tools to be used in conjunction with self-help methods, lifestyle changes, and other complementary therapies rather than stand-alone treatments. Since every person's experience with fibromyalgia is different, the treatment strategy should be customised for each patient.

In summary, interventional therapies such spinal cord stimulation, nerve blocks, and trigger point injections may be helpful in the management of fibromyalgia symptoms. They should be taken into account as a component of an all-encompassing treatment strategy, though, as they do carry certain hazards. We can provide fibromyalgia patients the tools they need to find relief and reclaim their lives by investigating a range of therapeutic alternatives, including interventional therapies.

Chapter 3: Holistic Approaches to Fibromyalgia Management

Nutrition and Diet

The influence of foods that cause inflammation is one of the most important things to comprehend about diet and fibromyalgia. With fibromyalgia, inflammation is a regular occurrence. Certain foods can aggravate these inflammatory processes, making pain and discomfort worse. Processed foods, refined sugars, trans fats, and highly processed vegetable oils are examples of foods that cause inflammation. These meals have the potential to set off a chain reaction of inflammation in the body, exacerbating symptoms and making fibromyalgia management even more difficult.

Adopting a balanced diet that emphasises lowering inflammation and boosting general health and well-being is essential to addressing this problem. A range of nutrient-dense foods, such as fruits, vegetables, whole grains, lean meats, and healthy fats, make up a balanced diet. These healthful foods offer the antioxidants and nutrients the body needs to promote the body's natural healing processes and reduce inflammation.

For those who have fibromyalgia, there are particular dietary guidelines that can be especially helpful in addition to maintaining a balanced diet. Increasing the amount of anti-inflammatory items in the diet is one such suggestion. These foods include leafy greens (like spinach and kale), nuts and seeds (like flaxseeds and walnuts), fatty fish (such salmon, mackerel, and sardines), and berries (such as blueberries and strawberries). Omega-3 fatty acids, antioxidants, and other nutrients with demonstrated anti-inflammatory effects can be found in abundance in these meals.

In addition, it's critical to take care of any possible nutritional deficiencies that can be causing symptoms of fibromyalgia. Patients with fibromyalgia frequently have shortages in magnesium, vitamin D, and B vitamins. While vitamin D is vital for immune system performance and general bone health, magnesium is essential for both muscle relaxation and pain control. B vitamins help the neurological system and energy generation, which are both frequently impacted by fibromyalgia. Thus, making sure you're getting enough of these nutrients via diet or supplements will help with symptom management.

The connection between gut health and symptoms is another dietary factor to take into account for fibromyalgia patients. Recent studies point to a connection between fibromyalgia and gut health, with changes in gut bacteria possibly influencing the intensity of symptoms. Consuming a diet high in fiber—found in fruits, vegetables, whole grains, and legumes—is crucial for maintaining a healthy gut. Furthermore, including foods that have undergone fermentation, such kefir, kimchi, sauerkraut, and yoghurt, can supply healthy probiotics that support the gut microbiota's restoration to equilibrium.

In addition to diet, maintaining adequate water is essential for managing fibromyalgia. Being dehydrated can make symptoms like exhaustion and muscular soreness worse, so it's critical to stay well hydrated all day. Consuming meals high in water content, like fruits and vegetables, can help maintain overall hydration levels in addition to drinking water.

Although following some dietary guidelines can help manage the symptoms of fibromyalgia, it's vital to keep in mind that each person is different and that what works for one may not work for another. It's critical to pay attention to how various meals and dietary practises affect your symptoms and to listen to your body. Maintaining a food journal can help you spot trends and triggers, which will help you manage your symptoms and customise your diet.

In summary, diet and nutrition are very important in controlling the symptoms of fibromyalgia. People with fibromyalgia can significantly improve their overall quality of life by focusing on lowering inflammation, adopting anti-inflammatory foods, correcting dietary shortages, supporting gut health, and staying hydrated. Always remember that before making any big dietary changes, you should speak with a medical expert or a qualified dietitian. They can offer individualised advice that is catered to your unique requirements. By working together and utilising a multidisciplinary approach, we can enable those who suffer with fibromyalgia to take charge of their health and enhance their life quality.

Sleep Hygiene and Relaxation Techniques

A crucial element of our general health and wellbeing is sleep. Sleep is when our bodies regenerate and restore themselves. However, getting a good night's sleep might be difficult for people who have fibromyalgia. Many patients commonly experience non-restorative sleep, frequent nighttime awakenings, or insomnia. Fibromyalgia symptoms are made worse by poor sleep, which results in greater pain, exhaustion, and impaired cognitive function.

Developing healthy sleep hygiene practises is essential to enhancing the quality of your slumber. A collection of behaviours and habits that support sound sleep is referred to as sleep hygiene. You may create a relaxing and sleep-friendly environment by adhering to these suggestions. Now let's explore some useful advice that will help you become an expert in good sleep hygiene.

Setting up a regular sleep pattern is one of the first steps to improved sleep hygiene. This entails setting a consistent bedtime and wake-up time every day, including on the weekends. You can better control your body's internal clock and facilitate natural sleep and wakefulness by adhering to a regular sleep schedule. Aim for seven to nine hours of sleep per night, making sure you leave adequate time for relaxation and recuperation.

It's also essential to create a sleep-friendly environment. It should be silent, dark, and cold in your bedroom. To filter out distracting outside noise, think about purchasing white noise generators, blackout curtains, or earplugs. Verify the comfort and support of your pillows and mattress. Try out a variety of pillows and mattress toppers to see which is most comfortable for you. You should also avoid using electronics in your bedroom because the blue light they create can disrupt your regular sleep-wake cycle.

It's critical to unwind before bed and let your body know when it's time to sleep. Take a warm bath, read a book, or practise relaxation techniques—a topic we will cover later in this chapter—to help you unwind. In the hours before bed, stay away from bright lights and stimulating activities as these can make it harder for you to fall asleep.

Establishing a nightly schedule can assist in preparing your body for sleep. Include things that encourage you to unwind and let you know when it's time to go to sleep. This can be journaling, doing some light stretching, or taking up a soothing pastime. Try a variety of things to see what personally calms and relaxes you.

Keeping up a healthy diet and exercise routine is also essential for proper sleep hygiene. Alcohol, nicotine, and caffeine should not be consumed right before bed since they can interfere with your sleep cycles. Rather, choose a light snack high in tryptophan, which is the building block for the chemicals melatonin and serotonin, which control sleep. Tryptophan-rich foods include dairy, nuts, seeds, and turkey.

Make exercise a regular part of your day, but try to finish your activity a few hours or earlier than when you go to bed. Exercise has been demonstrated to lessen fibromyalgia symptoms and enhance the quality of sleep. On the other hand, exercising too soon before bed might heighten awareness and cause difficulty falling asleep. Try out a variety of exercises to see what suits you the most, whether it's swimming, yoga, or walking.

Relaxation methods are crucial for controlling fibromyalgia symptoms and encouraging sound sleep in addition to good sleep hygiene. These methods aid in stress relief, mental clarity, and physical relaxation readiness. Let's look at some efficient relaxation methods that you might use on a regular basis.

Exercises involving deep breathing are an easy yet effective technique to promote relaxation. You can trigger your body's natural relaxation response by paying attention to your breath and taking slow, deep breaths. Close your eyes, find a comfortable posture, and take a deep breath through your nostrils while contracting your diaphragm. After holding your breath for a few while, gently release it through your mouth. Repeat this numerous times, letting your breathing become rhythmic and slow.

Another useful method for encouraging relaxation and lowering muscle tension is progressive muscle relaxation. Beginning at your toes and working your way up to your head, begin by tensing and then relaxing each muscle group in your body. Hold the tension you're creating in each muscle group for a short while before letting go of it. Allow any tension or stress to dissipate as you focus on the feelings of relaxation.

Using your imagination to conjure up a serene and comforting mental image is a technique known as guided imagery. Look find a peaceful, cosy spot to sit or lie down. Shut your eyes and picture yourself in a calm and peaceful setting. Envision every aspect of this location—the sights, sounds, and scents—and give yourself permission to lose yourself in the moment. Observe how your body and mind begin to calm down as you immerse yourself in your surroundings.

For encouraging relaxation and enhancing the quality of your sleep, mindfulness exercises and meditation are also quite helpful. By concentrating your attention on the here and now, you can cultivate mindfulness and emotional and mental detachment. Set aside some time every day to sit motionless and pay attention to your thoughts, feelings, and breathing. You will develop inner serenity and calmness over time, which will have a beneficial effect on your sleeping habits.

I've included useful advice and methods for enhancing sleep hygiene and introducing relaxing techniques into your everyday routine in this subchapter. You can feel more general well-being, improve the quality of your sleep, and lessen the symptoms of fibromyalgia by making sleep a priority and putting these ideas into practise. Keep in mind that it could take some time to form new routines and determine what suits you the best. Have self-compassion and faith in the process. You can become an expert in both relaxation and sleep hygiene, which are essential skills for managing your fibromyalgia.

Stress Management and Mindfulness

I genuinely think that the mind-body link plays a part in managing fibromyalgia. Stress is known to affect the body in both physical and psychological ways. Our bodies release the hormone cortisol in reaction to stress, which controls how we react to stresses. This stress response is intensified and extended in fibromyalgia patients, which exacerbates pain and other symptoms. Stress can also damage the immune system, interfere with cognitive function, and interfere with sleep habits, all of which can add to the complexity of fibromyalgia.

Breathing exercises, meditation, and mindfulness are effective methods for helping people with fibromyalgia control stress and how it affects their symptoms. Specifically, mindfulness is the practise of paying attention to and accepting the present moment without passing judgement. People with fibromyalgia can become more aware of their bodies and learn to manage the pain and discomfort they experience by practising mindfulness.

I suggest choosing a peaceful, cosy spot where you may sit or lie down to begin practising mindfulness. Start by focusing on your breathing and the sensation of air entering and leaving your body. You can become aware of new feelings, ideas, or bodily sensations. Simply notice them objectively rather than getting sucked into them, then shift your attention back to your breathing. You can become more at ease and be able to react to pressures in a more composed way by engaging in this activity.

Another effective method for managing stress in people with fibromyalgia is meditation. It entails narrowing one's focus and blocking off the constant flow of ideas that usually fill our minds. Numerous studies have demonstrated the benefits of meditation, including its ability to lower stress, ease pain, promote better sleep, and increase general wellbeing. There are a variety of meditation techniques, including body scan, loving-kindness, and guided meditation. You can discover which meditation technique most resonates with you by investigating several approaches.

Stress can be immediately managed with easy-to-use yet powerful breathing exercises. Breathing deeply and slowly can help to soothe the nervous system and trigger the relaxation response. One method I frequently suggest is diaphragmatic breathing. Put one hand on your chest and the other on your abdomen to begin. Inhale deeply through your nose, feeling your abdomen rise as air fills your lungs. As you slowly release the breath through your mouth, feel your belly drop back down. For a few minutes, repeat this practise while concentrating just on your breathing.

It is essential to include regular self-care activities in your daily routine in addition to these routines. There are many various ways to practise self-care, based on your interests and preferences. It could be doing things you enjoy, like going on adventures, taking up a hobby, or spending time with close friends and family. It might also involve maintaining your physical well-being with consistent exercise, a healthy diet, and enough sleep. You are providing yourself with the means and resources to enhance your general well-being and effectively manage stress by making self-care a priority.

Recognizing psychology's contribution to the treatment of fibromyalgia is also crucial. Chronic sickness and pain have a profound psychological impact that should not be undervalued. A lot of people who have fibromyalgia feel depressed, anxious, frustrated, and even melancholy. Developing coping mechanisms and addressing the emotional components of having fibromyalgia can be greatly aided by seeking assistance from a certified counsellor or therapist who specialises in chronic pain.

One form of therapy that has had encouraging outcomes in the management of fibromyalgia is cognitive-behavioral therapy (CBT). Its main goal is to help you recognise harmful thought patterns and swap them out for more adaptive and good ones. CBT can assist people in redefining how they view their symptoms, learning useful coping mechanisms, and cultivating a more balanced way of living.

Finally, I think that managing fibromyalgia requires a complete strategy. Apart from stress management strategies and psychological assistance, additional factors including healthy eating, consistent exercise, and sufficient sleep are crucial for symptom treatment. A comprehensive strategy that is customised to each person's needs can be obtained by working with a group of professionals from various health and wellness domains.

In conclusion, stress can worsen fibromyalgia symptoms and increase the difficulty of managing the condition. People with fibromyalgia can adopt stress-reduction strategies including breathing exercises, mindfulness, and meditation to help them feel more at ease and manage their symptoms more effectively. Furthermore, creating a thorough management plan that takes into account every facet of health and wellbeing and treating the psychological components of fibromyalgia through treatment can greatly enhance the quality of life for those who have the condition. By using the mind-body link to its full potential, people can manage their chronic disease and regain control over their life by learning to live with fibromyalgia.

Complementary Therapies for Fibromyalgia

Massage Therapy:

Massage therapy is one of the most well-known and often used complementary therapies for fibromyalgia. As a physician and health and wellness coach, I often suggest massage therapy to my patients as an integral element of their overall care strategy for fibromyalgia.

The soft tissues of the body, such as the muscles, tendons, ligaments, and connective tissues, are worked on during massage therapy. In massage treatment, a variety of techniques are employed, including trigger point therapy, deep tissue massage, and Swedish massage. Each method has advantages of its own and, depending on the patient's symptoms and preferences, may be more or less appropriate for fibromyalgia sufferers.

Numerous studies have demonstrated the potential advantages of massage therapy for fibromyalgia sufferers. It has been shown to primarily relieve pain and ease tense muscles. For fibromyalgia patients who have persistent discomfort and tight muscles, this is particularly crucial. Enhancing blood flow to the afflicted areas with massage therapy facilitates healing and relaxation.

Massage therapy has been demonstrated to help fibromyalgia sufferers sleep better in addition to relieving pain. Patients with fibromyalgia frequently have sleep difficulties like insomnia or restless legs syndrome. Massage therapy can lower stress levels and encourage relaxation, which helps improve sleep quality and increase wakefulness.

In addition, massage therapy can lessen the symptoms of anxiety and despair in fibromyalgia sufferers. One's mental and emotional health can suffer when they have a chronic illness like fibromyalgia. The whole sense of happiness and wellbeing of a patient can be significantly impacted by the soft touch and human connection that massage therapy offers.

It's crucial to remember that massage treatment may not be appropriate for everyone and may have certain drawbacks. People who have certain medical issues, including deep vein thrombosis or skin infections, for example, might need to avoid massage therapy or get permission from their doctor first. Furthermore, some fibromyalgia sufferers may discover that the pressure used during a massage is too great or uncomfortable, in which case they should look into different massage techniques or lessen the pressure.

Chiropractic Care:

Chiropractic treatment is another complementary therapy that may be helpful for people with fibromyalgia. The primary goals of chiropractic care are the identification, management, and avoidance of conditions affecting the musculoskeletal system, especially the spine. In order to enhance alignment and lessen pain and dysfunction, chiropractors move the spine and other joints in the body using manual adjustment techniques.

Studies have indicated that receiving chiropractic care can help fibromyalgia sufferers with pain management and function enhancement. Chiropractic adjustments can relieve nerve pressure and ease musculoskeletal tension by realigning the spine and restoring normal joint function. This may lead to better range of motion along with less discomfort and stiffness.

Furthermore, chiropractic adjustments can assist fibromyalgia sufferers get better quality sleep. A more balanced and calm condition of the body can be attained with the aid of spinal adjustments, which can improve sleep. Furthermore, chiropractic adjustments can ease tension and stress, both of which can aggravate fibromyalgia sufferers' inability to sleep.

It's crucial to understand that while some fibromyalgia sufferers may benefit from chiropractic care, this may not be the case or helpful for everyone. Seeking advice from a licenced and skilled chiropractor with experience in treating fibromyalgia sufferers is crucial. Furthermore, people who suffer from specific medical disorders, such osteoporosis or spinal cord compression, might need to avoid receiving adjustments from a chiropractor or get permission from their doctor.

Energy Healing:

An alternative form of therapy called energy healing seeks to clear the body of any blockages and bring it back into equilibrium. It is predicated on the idea that disorders of the body, mind, and spirit might result from disequilibrium in the body's energy fields. Qigong, acupuncture, and Reiki are a few examples of energy healing techniques.

Many fibromyalgia sufferers report benefits from energy healing techniques, despite the paucity of scientific evidence supporting their effectiveness. Energy healing modalities, like Reiki, entail the practitioner sending healing energy to the patient through gentle touch or hands hanging over the body.

Energy healing has been reported by some fibromyalgia sufferers to help ease pain and encourage relaxation. These exercises are said to support self-healing by rebalancing the body's energy fields. Moreover, energy healing methods can benefit an individual's mental and emotional health by lowering stress, anxiety, and depressive symptoms.

However, it's crucial to engage with a qualified and experienced practitioner and to approach energy healing with an open mind. Finding a practitioner who understands fibromyalgia and can customise energy healing sessions to meet the requirements and preferences of the patient is crucial.

Limitations of Complementary Therapies:

While complementary therapies have the potential to be very beneficial for people with fibromyalgia, it's critical to recognise their limitations. Complementary therapies are a useful tool to manage symptoms and improve general wellness, not a panacea for fibromyalgia.

It is important to keep in mind that each person is different, and what suits one person might not suit another. Finding the ideal mix of complementary therapies that would work best for a certain fibromyalgia sufferer may need some trial and error.

Additionally, it's critical to collaborate with licenced, experienced professionals who specialise in treating fibromyalgia patients. Throughout the course of treatment, these professionals can offer direction and support, enabling patients to make well-informed decisions regarding their health and welfare.

In conclusion, alternative therapies like energy healing, chiropractic adjustments, and massage therapy can be very helpful in managing fibromyalgia. These treatments may help with pain relief, lowering tense muscles, boosting general health, and improving quality of sleep. It is crucial to keep an open mind when pursuing these therapies, collaborate with licenced professionals, and acknowledge that they cannot treat fibromyalgia.

Chapter 4: Customizable Management Plans

Assessing Individual Needs

It is necessary to clarify a few essential concepts that will be used throughout this chapter before we get into the assessment procedure. First of all, anything pertaining to the body and how it functions is considered a physical necessity. This covers not only the degree of pain and symptoms but also other factors including energy levels, activity tolerance, and sleep habits. Conversely, psychological and mental health are included in emotional needs. Stress levels, mood swings, anxiety, and sadness are all included in this. Last but not least, lifestyle variables are the routines, habits, and external circumstances that go into daily life and might affect your general health. This covers one's food, routine, employment, interpersonal connections, and social support.

An essential part of managing fibromyalgia is evaluating your physical demands. It entails assessing your pain threshold, symptoms, and how they affect your day-to-day activities. You can keep a pain diary to record your symptoms and pain levels over time, which can help you become more aware of your physical demands. You will be able to track any changes in your condition and recognise trends and triggers as a result. Furthermore, by using body maps to identify pain and discomfort spots, you can better explain your symptoms to your medical staff.

In order to effectively manage fibromyalgia, it is as crucial to understand your emotional needs. It is commonly recognised that fibromyalgia affects mental health in addition to its physical manifestations. You can find any emotional stressors or triggers that might make your symptoms worse by evaluating your emotional needs. To measure your levels of anxiety and sadness, you can utilise questionnaires like the Generalized Anxiety Disorder (GAD-7) and Patient Health Questionnaire (PHQ-9). With the use of these resources, you may improve your comprehension of your mental health and receive the right guidance when seeking the necessary support.

The way one lives affects how one manages their fibromyalgia. Evaluating your way of life enables you to pinpoint any routines or behaviours that might be exacerbating your symptoms or impeding your capacity to successfully manage the illness. Assessing your nutrition and diet is a good place to start because some foods might exacerbate symptoms or cause inflammatory reactions. Maintaining a food journal and observing how your body reacts to various foods will assist you in determining any dietary adjustments that could enhance your general health.

Controlling your everyday activities and stress levels is crucial for managing fibromyalgia, in addition to food. You can modify your habits by determining which activities might be putting too much strain or stress on your body. In a similar vein, becoming aware of your stress levels and identifying constructive coping strategies can greatly enhance your general wellbeing. To determine your current stress level and probable sources of stress in your life, use stress assessment tools.

Understanding your unique demands is a continuous process rather than a one-time event. Your condition could change over time, so it's critical to frequently review and analyse your needs. You can make sure that your management plan continues to match your changing demands by using the self-assessment tools and conducting regular self-checks.

In summary, determining your unique needs is an essential first step toward successfully managing fibromyalgia. You can design a tailored management plan that takes into account your particular circumstances by gaining an awareness of your lifestyle, emotional, and physical characteristics. This chapter's self-assessment tools and questionnaires can assist you in gaining perspective, directing you toward the right kind of support, and helping you change your way of living. Recall that treating fibromyalgia is a multifaceted process that necessitates a thorough comprehension of your unique requirements.

Creating a Personalized Management Plan

Fibromyalgia can be difficult to live with because of its fluctuating pain and tiredness thresholds and erratic symptoms. You may, however, reclaim control over your life and enhance your general well-being by managing your disease proactively. To do this, you must design a customised management plan that takes into account your particular requirements and objectives.

Setting goals is the first stage in developing an individualised management strategy. When it comes to managing your fibromyalgia, what are your goals? Are you want to feel less discomfort, get better sleep, or have more energy? Or maybe you want to do things that make you happy and fulfilled? Whatever your objectives, it's critical to know exactly what you hope to accomplish.

Setting priorities for your goals is crucial once you've defined them. Prioritizing your objectives will enable you to concentrate your efforts and use your resources wisely. For instance, if alleviating pain is your main concern, you can decide to give pain management-specific therapies and treatments top priority.

It's time to prioritise your objectives and then develop an action plan that combines holistic and medical methods. Because fibromyalgia is a complicated disorder, managing it requires a multifaceted strategy. Wholesome strategies like lifestyle changes, complementary therapies, and self-care practises are just as vital for managing symptoms as pharmaceuticals and medical interventions.

Medical Approaches:

By including medical techniques in your treatment plan, you can alleviate symptoms and enhance your general well-being. You can find an efficient treatment plan by collaborating closely with your healthcare team, which may include a physical therapist, rheumatologist, and pain expert.

Medication: Your doctor may recommend medication to treat pain, enhance sleep, or lessen exhaustion, depending on your individual symptoms. Medication for fibromyalgia frequently consists of antidepressants, sleep aids, and pain medicines.

Physical therapy: Enhancing muscle strength, flexibility, and general physical function can be achieved with physical therapy. An exercise regimen customised to your requirements and capabilities by your physical therapist can help reduce pain and increase your vitality.

Holistic Approaches:

Treating the full person—their physical, mental, and emotional well-being—is the main goal of holistic therapies. Although there may not be a cure for fibromyalgia, these methods can greatly lessen symptoms and improve your quality of life in general.

Lifestyle modifications: You can significantly reduce the symptoms of fibromyalgia by making specific changes to your daily routine and habits. This can entail creating a regular sleep pattern, engaging in stress-reduction activities, and adding mild exercise regimens like tai chi or yoga.

Alternative therapies: A lot of people with fibromyalgia find relief with complementary therapies including massage, acupuncture, and chiropractic adjustments. These treatments can ease discomfort, enhance relaxation, and improve sleep.

Self-care techniques: Taking care of oneself is crucial to controlling fibromyalgia. This could entail engaging in self-help activities to lower stress and enhance emotional wellbeing, like deep breathing exercises, meditation, or mindfulness. It may also entail introducing enjoyable and unwinding activities into your routine, such taking up a hobby or going outside.

Coping strategies: The difficulties of having fibromyalgia can be overcome with the use of useful coping mechanisms. This can entail learning how to pace oneself by striking a balance between activity and rest, going to support groups or therapy sessions, and asking for help from people who are aware of your disease.

Through the integration of medical approaches and holistic solutions, a complete care plan that takes into account every facet of your fibromyalgia can be developed. Recall that developing a customised management plan is a continuous process that changes in response to your demands and objectives. It's critical to frequently evaluate your progress, make changes as needed, and enlist the help of your loved ones and your healthcare team.

To sum up, developing a customised management plan is an essential first step toward managing your fibromyalgia. This entails establishing your objectives, ranking them, and incorporating holistic and medical methods into your strategy. Regaining control over your life and enhancing your general well-being can be achieved by adopting a proactive approach and utilising a variety of strategies and techniques. Recall that you are not alone on this road and that you can overcome fibromyalgia by finding the support and tools you need.

Adapting Strategies for Daily Life

1. Overcoming Challenges:

There are several difficulties associated with having fibromyalgia, both psychological and physical. But it's important to keep in mind that you are not travelling alone. It can really help to surround yourself with a network of friends, family, and medical professionals who are supportive.

Fatigue is one of the biggest issues fibromyalgia sufferers deal with. Even the easiest chores can appear onerous because of this overpowering fatigue. It's critical to prioritise your tasks according to your energy levels and arrange your activities in order to overcome this difficulty. Ensure that you pace yourself and divide your work into smaller, more doable portions. Pay attention to your body's cues and take breaks when required.

Another essential component of overcoming obstacles in daily life is learning to manage discomfort. Through some trial and error, the ideal combination of pain management strategies must be determined. Seeking advice from your healthcare professional is crucial as you consider different choices including prescription drugs, physical therapy, acupuncture, or complementary therapies like yoga and meditation.

2. Managing Flare-Ups:

Unfortunately, flare-ups are a common occurrence for fibromyalgia sufferers. Your everyday routine may be disturbed by these brief, powerful outbursts, which may also make you feel powerless. But, if you have a strategy in place, you can deal with flare-ups when they happen.

Determine your triggers first. To monitor your symptoms and record any trends or activities that seem to exacerbate them, keep a notebook. This will lessen the possibility of a flare-up by assisting you in identifying and avoiding triggers.

It's critical to establish a self-care regimen that you can adhere to during flare-ups. The main goals of this regimen should be pain management, relaxation, and rest. To help reduce your symptoms during a flare-up, incorporate methods like deep breathing exercises, mindfulness meditation, heat or cold therapy, and mild stretching. Never forget that it's critical to customise your self-care regimen to your own requirements and preferences.

Having an understanding support system that can relate to your condition is essential to managing flare-ups. To get emotional support and advice from those who have gone through similar experiences, get in touch with support groups, online forums, or seek professional assistance. Creating a network of sympathetic people can help you get through the difficult times.

3. Staying Motivated:

It takes commitment and tenacity to achieve better health, which can be especially difficult when one has fibromyalgia. But maintaining your motivation is essential to moving forward and accomplishing your objectives.

An essential component of maintaining motivation is setting reasonable goals. To begin, list the aspects of your life that you would like to better control or enhance. It might be getting more exercise, making better dietary choices, or learning useful stress-reduction strategies. Divide these objectives into more manageable segments, and acknowledge each accomplishment as you proceed.

Keeping an optimistic outlook is crucial to being motivated. It's critical to prevent negative thoughts and self-doubt from taking over. Instead, pay attention to the advancements and enhancements you have already experienced. Remain connected to the good things in your life, such the moments you spend with your loved ones, the hobbies you enjoy, or the things that make you happy. Having an optimistic outlook will help you advance in your quest for improved health.

Reevaluating and adjusting your strategies on a regular basis is also essential to maintaining motivation. Make adjustments to your routines and approaches as you gain more understanding of your body and what functions best for you. Continue to be receptive to new ideas and eager to try things out until you figure out what works best for you. Accept the voyage as a chance for personal development and exploration.

4. Conclusion:

To effectively manage your fibromyalgia, you must be committed, patient, and flexible in your approach. Through conquering these obstacles, controlling relapses, and maintaining your drive, you can change your day-to-day existence and enhance your general health.

Never forget that you are not travelling alone. Join support groups, ask your healthcare practitioner for assistance, and surround yourself with compassionate people. Accept the power of self-care and include it into your daily schedule, customising it to meet your individual requirements. To stay motivated, make sure your goals are reasonable, have an optimistic outlook, and periodically review your tactics.

Even though having fibromyalgia can come with its share of challenges, it does not define you. You can find empowerment and take back control of your life if you apply the appropriate techniques and make a commitment to your wellbeing. Breathe deeply, accept the difficulties, and set off on this life-changing adventure with courage and resiliency. I know you can learn to manage your fibromyalgia, and this book will be your reliable guide.

Tracking Progress and Making Adjustments

This chapter stresses the significance of monitoring development and modifying the management strategy as necessary. It talks about how to maximise results by engaging in self-reflection, self-monitoring, and professional advice. I have personally experienced the transformational effect of these practises as a medical practitioner and health and wellness coach.

It takes more than merely documenting physical symptoms or flare-ups to track improvement. It is far more than that. It entails a thorough evaluation of all the facets of a person's life that may have an impact on their general wellbeing and fibromyalgia symptoms. This entails monitoring trends in eating habits, sleep, exercise, stress, and mental health. Through the use of contemporary technology or a thorough notebook, people can start to see trends and triggers that are related to their symptoms.

In this process, self-reflection is a very useful tool. It invites people to delve deeply into their feelings, ideas, and perspectives related to their experience with fibromyalgia. By engaging in introspective activities like writing, mindfulness, and meditation, people can find underlying stressors, unhelpful thought patterns, and emotional disturbances that might be influencing their symptoms. People can then start making the required changes to their management strategy by illuminating these internal mechanisms.

An additional crucial component of tracking development is self-monitoring. This entails routinely evaluating one's degree of weariness, pain, and bodily symptoms. People who regularly track these facets of daily life are able to recognise patterns and variations in their symptoms. Then, based on this information, their treatment plan can be modified.

But it's crucial to keep in mind that monitoring development and implementing changes shouldn't be done separately. It is imperative to seek professional counsel, since healthcare providers may provide invaluable insights and expertise. I work directly with my patients as a medical doctor and health and wellness coach to help them through this journey. Together, we examine the data, spot patterns, and modify the treatment strategy. Through the integration of their personal experiences with my medical expertise, we can devise a complete care strategy customised to meet their specific requirements.

The care of fibromyalgia must be approached holistically in order to maximise results. This entails taking into account social, psychological, and emotional elements of the illness in addition to its physical manifestations, as they may have an impact on how severe symptoms are. Adopting a multidisciplinary strategy, I put together a group of professionals from different areas of health and wellbeing to provide my patients a holistic approach to their treatment.

Modifications to one's lifestyle are crucial for monitoring development and making improvements. People can actively control their symptoms by making modifications to their nutrition, exercise routine, stress reduction techniques, and sleep hygiene. These adjustments can be made to target particular triggers and symptom patterns that self-reflection and self-monitoring have identified.

Psychological treatments and counselling are useful instruments on this path. Through addressing the psychological and emotional elements of fibromyalgia, people can cultivate a positive outlook, learn coping mechanisms, and become more resilient. Improved results and a higher standard of living can be attained by methods including mindfulness-based stress reduction (MBSR), cognitive-behavioral therapy (CBT), and relaxation exercises.

It's also critical to include complementary and alternative methods of self-care. These can include, among other things, massage treatment, yoga, tai chi, and acupuncture. People can discover more help and symptom relief by investigating these many options. These methods are adaptable to the preferences of the individual, guaranteeing a comprehensive and unique approach to managing fibromyalgia.

Finally, coping mechanisms and self-help approaches are crucial instruments for monitoring development and adjusting course. These methods enable patients to actively engage in their treatment plan and take charge of their own health. Through the use of skills like self-compassion exercises, pacing activities, and stress management approaches, people with fibromyalgia can face their condition head-on and with resiliency.

To sum up, monitoring development and making modifications are critical elements of successful fibromyalgia treatment. By use of introspection, self-observation, and obtaining expert advice, people can enhance their results and elevate their standard of living. People can take control of their fibromyalgia journey and discover newfound hope and empowerment along the way by adopting a holistic approach that incorporates lifestyle modifications, counselling and psychology-related techniques, self-care alternative and complementary techniques, as well as self-help techniques and coping strategies.

Chapter 5: Nurturing Emotional Well-being

Understanding the Emotional Impact of Fibromyalgia

We must first get a deeper grasp of fibromyalgia in order to fully comprehend the condition's emotional impact. Fatigue, sensitivity in particular body parts, and diffuse musculoskeletal pain are the hallmarks of fibromyalgia, a chronic illness. A person's quality of life may be significantly impacted by these symptoms, which can be incapacitating. Nonetheless, it's critical to understand that fibromyalgia affects the mind and emotions in addition to the body.

There are many difficulties associated with having chronic pain and exhaustion. A typical emotional challenge faced by people with fibromyalgia is feeling bereaved and grieving. Suffering from persistent pain and exhaustion can make it difficult to go about everyday tasks, engage in hobbies, and keep relationships together. This loss of capability may cause annoyance, rage, or depression.

Additionally, people with fibromyalgia may find it challenging to schedule and engage in activities due to the erratic nature of their symptoms, which can result in social disengagement and a sense of loneliness. It might be difficult to make commitments or interact socially when there is a worry of an unexpected flare-up of pain or exhaustion. Feelings of depression and loneliness may eventually result from this seclusion.

The psychological components of fibromyalgia symptoms are frequently intricate and multidimensional. Mood problems such as anxiety and sadness can arise from the imbalance of neurotransmitters in the brain caused by chronic pain. Furthermore, fibromyalgia sufferers may experience central sensitization, or an increased sensitivity to pain, which can worsen mental anguish.

One important aspect of fibromyalgia is the mind-body link. Studies have indicated that fibromyalgia symptoms might be exacerbated or triggered by stress and emotional trauma. Our bodies release the stress hormone cortisol during times of stress, which can exacerbate inflammation and pain sensitivity. Long-term stress can also cause muscle tension and a lower pain threshold, which exacerbates the symptoms of fibromyalgia.

Moreover, fibromyalgia affects people's emotional health in ways that go beyond the condition's physical manifestations. Constantly battling with discomfort and exhaustion can cause a person to lose their sense of self and suffer from low self-esteem. Many fibromyalgia sufferers experience emotions of powerlessness and purposelessness as a result of feeling as though they no longer have control over their bodies or their lives.

My objective as a medical professional and health and wellness coach is to offer a comprehensive method of managing fibromyalgia. In my opinion, treating the psychological effects of fibromyalgia is equally as crucial as treating the physical manifestations of the condition. Through comprehension of the psychological elements that contribute to the symptoms of fibromyalgia and the mind-body link, we may create useful coping mechanisms and resources to help patients take back control of their life.

Making lifestyle changes is one of the most important strategies for coping with the emotional effects of fibromyalgia. This entails introducing stress-reduction methods into regular activities, such as mindfulness, meditation, and relaxation exercises. These methods can aid in lowering the body's levels of stress-related chemicals and encourage tranquilly and wellbeing.

Using counselling and psychology-related practises is a crucial part of controlling the emotional impact. Therapy can offer a secure and encouraging setting where people can examine their feelings, learn stress management techniques, and build coping mechanisms. For those suffering from fibromyalgia, cognitive-behavioral therapy (CBT) is especially helpful since it can help recognise and address harmful thought patterns and beliefs that fuel emotional distress.

Alternative and complementary therapies can be helpful in addressing the emotional burden of fibromyalgia in addition to standard therapies. Methods like yoga, massage treatment, and acupuncture can ease pain, ease tension, and encourage calmness. These methods not only ease physical discomfort but also instil harmony and balance in the body and mind.

Additionally crucial resources for managing emotional well-being for people with fibromyalgia are self-help skills and coping strategies. This entails engaging in self-care activities including hobbies, preserving social links, and establishing reasonable objectives. Additionally, people can save energy and avoid pain and tiredness flare-ups by learning to pace themselves and prioritise self-care.

In summary, effective care of fibromyalgia requires a knowledge of the emotional consequences of the chronic condition. In addition to its physical effects, fibromyalgia has a negative impact on a person's emotional health. By identifying the intricate psychological elements that underlie the symptoms of fibromyalgia and investigating the mind-body link, we may create all-encompassing plans and networks of support to assist people in taking back control of their life. Despite their obstacles, people with fibromyalgia can discover empowerment and increased mental well-being through lifestyle modifications, counselling and psychology-related practises, alternative and complementary therapies, and self-help tactics.

Coping With Stress and Anxiety

Stress, whether it originates internally from unfavourable thoughts or externally from demands at work, causes physiological reactions in the body that can exacerbate the symptoms of fibromyalgia. On the other side, anxiety thrives on ambiguity and a dread of the unknown, which can leave people feeling uneasy all the time and exacerbate their pain. You can better manage your fibromyalgia by escaping the cycle of stress and worry by comprehending these links and putting healthy coping mechanisms into practise.

Relaxation techniques are a vital component of managing stress and anxiety. The negative impacts of stress can be offset by consciously triggering the body's relaxation response. Effective techniques for inducing this reaction include progressive muscle relaxation, deep breathing exercises, visualisation, and meditation. During deep breathing exercises, you should take slow, deep breaths while paying attention to how your breath enters and exits your body. Let your body let go of any stress and negativity as you exhale. Progressive muscle relaxation, on the other hand, encourages a feeling of release and serenity by first tensing and then relaxing various muscle groups. Your mind and body may relax and calm down by using guided images and visualisations to take you to a serene state. By practising mindfulness or focused attention meditation, you can develop awareness and acceptance of your thoughts and sensations without passing judgement. Meditation helps you to centre yourself in the present now. You can lessen the effect of stress and worry on your fibromyalgia symptoms by adopting these relaxing techniques into your everyday routine.

A further effective method for managing stress and anxiety is by applying the concepts of cognitive-behavioral therapy (CBT). This method focuses on locating and disputing unfavourable ideas and attitudes that fuel tension and worry. You can obtain a more realistic and balanced perspective by looking at the data both in favour of and against these ideas. CBT can assist you in rephrasing your ideas and coming up with alternate, more optimistic interpretations, for instance, if you frequently find yourself catastrophizing about the future or expecting the worst. Furthermore, CBT equips you with useful abilities like assertiveness and problem-solving, enabling you to take charge of the circumstances that are causing you stress and worry. You can overcome the difficulties caused by fibromyalgia with a more upbeat and resilient mindset by consistently practising these behavioural and cognitive strategies.

Lifestyle changes are essential for controlling stress and anxiety in the setting of fibromyalgia, in addition to relaxation methods and cognitive behavioural therapy (CBT) concepts. It's critical to pay attention to your sleep patterns because getting too little sleep can lead to a marked increase in stress. To encourage restful and revitalising sleep, set up a regular sleep schedule, establish a relaxing nighttime ritual, and create an environment that is conducive to sleep. In addition to lowering stress, regular exercise that is catered to your unique requirements and restrictions releases endorphins, the body's natural opioids that can improve mood and lessen pain. Take part in the things that make you happy and fulfilled, whether they are artistic endeavours, hobbies, or relationships with loved ones. These changes to one's lifestyle promote wellbeing and a sense of purpose in addition to acting as stress and anxiety relievers.

The foundation of managing stress and anxiety in people with fibromyalgia is self-care. Prioritizing your mental, emotional, and physical health is crucial. This entails establishing limits and using the word "no" when appropriate. To give yourself the time and space to attend to your own needs, learn to assign duties and obligations. Take part in self-soothing and relaxation-promoting activities, such aromatherapy, warm baths, and massage therapy. Take care of your connections and look for assistance from people who can relate to and understand your experience. Keep in mind that there is power in community and that you are not alone in your fight.

Finally, in order to deal with stress and anxiety, it's critical to establish efficient coping mechanisms. For instance, keeping a journal gives you a therapeutic outlet and helps you process and let go of your feelings. Throughout the day, cultivate mindfulness by focusing on the here and now and establishing a connection with it. Make use of stress-reduction strategies like time management and organising to lessen overwhelm and boost output. Try out several complementary and alternative therapies, like yoga, acupuncture, and herbal supplements, to see what suits you the best. Always keep in mind that there is no one-size-fits-all method for handling stress and anxiety; instead, you must experiment until you find a strategy that works for your particular requirements and preferences.

To sum up, stress and worry are powerful enemies that can cause severe damage to people who have fibromyalgia. But with the appropriate tools, you can take back control and get your life back. You can lessen the negative effects of stress and anxiety on your fibromyalgia symptoms by implementing relaxation methods, cognitive-behavioral therapy concepts, and lifestyle changes into your everyday routine. Recall that stress reduction and self-care are essential elements of successful fibromyalgia management, enabling you to live a happy and meaningful life in spite of your obstacles. My honest wish is that the knowledge and techniques in this chapter may act as a beacon for you as you go toward being an expert with your fibromyalgia..

Overcoming Depression and Boosting Mood

Fibromyalgia and depression frequently coexist, producing a vicious cycle that can be very difficult to escape. It makes sense that having fibromyalgia would have an adverse effect on one's mental state, resulting in depressive, gloomy, and even hopeless feelings. This emotional load then feeds back into the physical manifestations of fibromyalgia, intensifying the pain cycle.

For patients and healthcare providers alike, realising this connection between depression and fibromyalgia is a crucial first step. By realising that depression is a legitimate comorbidity and not just a symptom of physical illness, we can confront the issue head-on and create opportunities for successful interventions.

Therapy is a very useful strategy for overcoming depression in the context of fibromyalgia. Individuals can examine their feelings, difficulties, and concerns in a safe and encouraging setting by participating in therapy. Counseling, whether through psychodynamic therapy, cognitive-behavioral therapy (CBT), or other evidence-based approaches, can assist patients in changing the way they think, handling stress, and creating useful coping strategies.

Building a support system and obtaining professional therapy are essential for overcoming depression. Making a connection with people who understand the special difficulties associated with having fibromyalgia can be quite empowering. Both in-person and virtual support groups give people the chance to talk about their experiences, develop empathy, and get insightful advice from people who genuinely know what they're going through. Whether it be friends, family, or other fibromyalgia warriors, having a strong support network can help reduce feelings of loneliness and offer a much-needed sense of understanding and belonging.

Self-help methods can be used to elevate mood and enhance emotional well-being, even though counselling and support groups provide vital direction and affirmation. These methods can be used independently as people figure out what suits them best, or in concert with expert supervision.

Exercise is one self-help method that has demonstrated encouraging benefits in the management of fibromyalgia and depression. Regular physical activity, such as yoga, tai chi, or low-impact workouts, can release endorphins, which are feel-good hormones that naturally elevate mood, in addition to helping with pain relief and improving physical functioning. Exercise should be started cautiously and increased in duration and intensity gradually to prevent aggravating the symptoms of fibromyalgia. An exercise regimen designed specifically for each person, taking into account their preferences and talents, can improve their general health.

Incorporating mindfulness and relaxation practises into one's everyday routine is another effective strategy. Being mindful entails focusing on and accepting the current situation without passing judgement. Deep breathing exercises, meditation, and even taking a soothing bath can help people manage their stress levels and anxiety, which makes it easier for them to deal with the difficulties that come with fibromyalgia and depression. Regular mindfulness practise can also help you become more self-aware and assist you in escaping harmful thought patterns.

It is noteworthy that controlling depression related to fibromyalgia might also benefit from the use of complementary and alternative therapies. The potential benefits of techniques like acupuncture, massage, and aromatherapy in encouraging relaxation, mood improvement, and pain reduction have made them more and more popular in recent years. Although the scientific data supporting the efficacy of these therapies for fibromyalgia is still developing, excellent outcomes reported by certain patients underscores the need of individualised and integrative methods.

Ultimately, it is critical to keep in mind that every person's road to overcome melancholy and improve mood is different. Finding the tactics that work for one person's unique needs and circumstances may need persistence, patience, and an open mind. What works for one person may not necessarily work for another. Creating a comprehensive strategy for managing fibromyalgia that takes into account mental, emotional, and physical health is essential for long-term success and a general increase in quality of life.

We have looked at the complex relationship between fibromyalgia and depression in this subchapter and have also discovered methods for improving mood and conquering depression. Through the use of self-help tactics, support networks, and treatment, people can overcome the obstacles that depression presents and take back control of their mental health. Even if the road may occasionally be challenging, it's important to keep in mind that there is hope and that, with enough effort, one may become master of both depression and fibromyalgia.

Cultivating Resilience and Self-Care

Although having fibromyalgia might frequently feel overwhelming, it's important to remember that our illness does not define who we are. The cornerstone of developing resilience in the face of these difficulties is self-compassion. It entails being kind, understanding, and accepting of ourselves instead of passing judgement or blaming ourselves for who we are not. We can change our perspective from one of self-blame to one of self-support and encouragement by practising self-compassion.

Recognizing and accepting our limits is the first step towards practising self-compassion. It's crucial to understand that fibromyalgia is not our fault when even the most basic chores seem difficult. It is imperative to let go of any guilt or shame we may be experiencing about our limits because we did not choose to have this illness. Rather, we should see these difficulties as chances to practise self-compassion and put our health first.

Another essential component of developing resilience and practising self-care when dealing with fibromyalgia is setting limits. It entails being aware of, respecting, and open about our emotional and physical boundaries with others around us. Some people may find this difficult since they frequently feel under pressure to put up with their discomfort and exhaustion in order to live up to others' expectations. Nonetheless, we are safeguarding our mental and physical well-being when we establish and uphold boundaries.

Saying no to commitments or activities that are above our current skills is one way to set boundaries. It could also entail giving up on projects that are too much for us or asking loved ones for assistance. Establishing boundaries teaches others how to best help us on our fibromyalgia journey while also emphasising our own well-being.

To overcome the challenges of fibromyalgia, it is essential to engage in activities that promote joy and well-being in addition to practising self-compassion and setting boundaries. Pleasurable activities can help lower pain perception, elevate mood, and promote general well-being, according to research. Finding happiness and pleasure in our daily lives serves as a counterbalance to any challenges our illness may present.

It takes a very personalised process to find things to do that make us happy and give us a sense of direction. It could entail experimenting with artistic mediums including writing, painting, or performing music. Exercises that are mild on the body, like tai chi or yoga, can help improve mental and physical health. Engaging in outdoor pursuits like hiking or gardening can foster a sense of renewal and tranquilly. Whatever it is, we must prioritise these things in our daily lives and make time for them.

To genuinely foster resilience and engage in self-care, these activities must be seen as continuous and dynamic. Our approach to resilience and self-care needs to be adaptive, just as fibromyalgia poses diverse obstacles. It's critical to keep trying out new coping mechanisms, looking for enjoyable hobbies, and reevaluating our boundaries when our requirements shift.

As a physician and health and wellness coach, I have personally witnessed the transforming effects of developing resilience and engaging in self-care when dealing with fibromyalgia difficulties. People are able to recover their sense of self and genuinely flourish in spite of their circumstances by using these techniques. I urge you to practise self-compassion, establish healthy boundaries, and partake in enjoyable and fulfilling activities. You are reclaiming your life and actively managing your fibromyalgia by doing this.

Chapter 6: Building a Supportive Network

Communicating With Loved Ones

Being self-aware is the first and most crucial stage in communicating. Spend some time getting to know your own wants, feelings, and constraints. You will be in a better position to communicate your experiences and problems to your loved ones if you have a clear grasp of them. By helping you differentiate between what is under your control and what is not, this self-awareness can also help you set reasonable expectations for both yourself and other people.

Expressing Needs:

It's critical to be upfront and honest about your wants when interacting with your loved ones. But when you're coping with the unpredictable and erratic symptoms of fibromyalgia, this can be difficult. To communicate your wants clearly:

1. Choose the right time and place: Look for a quiet, cosy spot where you can talk without being interrupted. This will establish a secure environment in which each party may communicate their ideas and emotions.

2. Be specific: Clearly state and express what you require. For instance, be more detailed about the symptoms you are having and how they are affecting you rather than just expressing, "I don't feel well."

3. Use "I" statements: Refrain from using accusatory or blaming words since this could make the other person defensive. Instead, describe your needs and feelings using "I" phrases. Say something like, "I need some more rest today since I feel overwhelmed and fatigued."

4. Provide examples: It can occasionally be challenging for other people to completely understand how fibromyalgia affects your day-to-day existence. Give concrete examples of how your symptoms interfere with your ability to carry out particular activities or engage in certain tasks. This can make fibromyalgia's severity and complexity more understandable to your loved ones.

Setting Boundaries:

You need to set limits if you want to keep your mental and physical health. Setting limits when those close to you do not fully comprehend or accept the limitations imposed by fibromyalgia can be difficult. The following advice will assist you in establishing and upholding appropriate boundaries:

1. Be assertive: Express your boundaries clearly, but do so in a kind and firm way. You are free to refuse requests and put your own needs first without feeling bad about it.

2. Educate your loved ones: Spend some time educating the people you care about about fibromyalgia. Distribute books, articles, or other instructional materials that succinctly and clearly describe the condition. With this understanding, they will be better able to recognise your limitations and modify their expectations.

3. Involve your loved ones in your treatment plan: Inspire your family members to take an active role in your treatment regimen. This may entail going to therapy sessions, support group meetings, or doctor's appointments together. Including them in your journey helps promote understanding and cooperation.

4. Practice self-compassion: There are moments when establishing and upholding boundaries might bring on guilt or a dread of disappointing other people. Remind yourself that taking care of yourself will make it easier for you to be there for your loved ones and that it is acceptable to put your health first.

Fostering Understanding and Empathy:

Establishing boundaries and communicating your needs are vital, but so is fostering an atmosphere of empathy and understanding in your relationships. The following are some methods to promote empathy and understanding:

1. Encourage communication: Provide a free-flowing, secure environment for your loved ones to share their opinions regarding your condition. Urge them to pose inquiries and attentively hear their viewpoint without passing judgement.

2. Practice active listening: As your loved ones express their ideas or worries, pay close attention to what they have to say. Even though they may not completely get your experience, be understanding and give them credit for their feelings. This promotes open conversation and a two-way understanding.

3. Provide educational resources: Give your loved ones access to educational materials that can give them a better understanding of fibromyalgia. Articles, books, movies, and support group gatherings may fall under this category.

4. Seek professional help: It might sometimes be advantageous for you and your loved ones to seek the advice of a therapist or counsellor. A specialist can offer methods and strategies for clear communication as well as support in overcoming obstacles.

Recall that developing better communication habits requires time and effort on the part of both parties. It is crucial to approach these discussions with tolerance, compassion, and an open mind. You can fortify the network of support people around you and enhance your connections by putting these tactics into practise.

The significance of self-care will be discussed in more detail in the upcoming chapter, along with a variety of complementary and alternative therapies that can be used to manage fibromyalgia symptoms. Watch this space for useful advice on how to put your physical and mental health first.

Seeking Professional Support

Let me stress again how crucial it is to put together a medical team that is knowledgeable on fibromyalgia. In this discipline, rheumatologists, pain management specialists, physical therapists, dietitians, and psychologists are among the sought-after practitioners. A comprehensive approach is necessary to treat the different aspects of fibromyalgia and how it affects your overall health.

Asking your primary care physician or other fibromyalgia patients for advice is one of the first steps in locating the ideal healthcare team. Referrals from friends and family can frequently offer important information about medical specialists who specialise in treating fibromyalgia. Furthermore, fibromyalgia-specific internet forums and support groups can be a goldmine of knowledge, connecting you with people who have had good results with specific medical specialists.

Asking the proper questions in the first session is important when contacting potential healthcare providers. This will enable you to evaluate their knowledge and comprehension of fibromyalgia and the recommended treatment modalities. Some important queries to think about could be:

1. Have you treated patients with fibromyalgia before?

2. What treatment options do you typically recommend for fibromyalgia management?

3. How do you approach the emotional and psychological aspects of fibromyalgia?

4. Are you familiar with integrative or complementary therapies that may benefit fibromyalgia patients?

Finding out the answers to these queries can help you assess the level of experience, philosophy, and suitability of the healthcare professional for your needs as a patient.

After your healthcare team is put together, good communication is essential to building a fruitful collaboration. The level of care you receive can be greatly impacted by establishing a relationship based on mutual respect, understanding, and candid communication. It is imperative that you take a strong stance in defending your demands and actively participate in your healthcare journey.

Making appointments in advance is one approach to enhance communication with your healthcare professionals. Making a note of the queries and issues you would like to discuss during the visit may be useful. This guarantees that you address all relevant areas of your health with your healthcare professional and that the conversation is fruitful.

It's critical to be honest and upfront about your symptoms, experiences, and any difficulties you may be having during consultations. Your healthcare professionals will be able to fully comprehend your situation with the help of honesty and clarity, which will enable them to customise treatment strategies just for you.

It is important to keep in mind that the people who administer your healthcare are not mind readers. It is crucial that you speak out if a treatment plan or medicine isn't working for you. You can investigate different solutions, tweaks, or modifications with your medical team in order to better manage your fibromyalgia symptoms. Recall that you have a voice and that you actively participate in your own care.

When you go to your doctor, keeping a notebook or symptom log can also be very helpful. Keep a journal of any changes you see in your symptoms, triggers, or patterns since these can offer important new perspectives on your illness. By providing your healthcare providers with this information, you may help them make more informed treatment decisions and identify areas that need more support or intervention.

As important as medical experts are in helping you manage your fibromyalgia, you also need to understand the importance of self-advocacy. The only person who truly knows your particular needs, experiences, and limitations is you, the patient. You can make sure that your voice and preferences are heard and appreciated by standing up for yourself.

Learning more about fibromyalgia is one way you can be an advocate for yourself. Being aware of the illness, its signs, and possible treatments gives you the power to choose your care with knowledge. With this knowledge, you will be able to take an active role in your own management and have meaningful conversations with your healthcare team.

Participating actively in fibromyalgia support groups or online forums can also provide a wealth of information and direction. Making connections with other fibromyalgia sufferers can give you a feeling of support, encourage a common understanding of the difficulties you have, and lead to the discovery of coping mechanisms that have been successful for other people. In trying times, these relationships can also offer emotional support.

As you embark on your quest for expert assistance, keep in mind that there isn't a single solution that works for everyone. Since each fibromyalgia patient is different, research and patience may be needed to choose the best healthcare team. Show yourself and the process some patience. Remind yourself that you are not alone in your struggle and that you can design a complete and unique plan for managing your fibromyalgia with the correct help, direction, and self-advocacy.

We shall examine the critical impact that lifestyle changes play in the management of fibromyalgia in the upcoming subchapter. We'll look at a variety of daily activities that can have a big impact on your fibromyalgia symptoms, from dietary adjustments to stress reduction methods. As we reveal the all-encompassing strategy for total fibromyalgia care, stay tuned.

Joining Support Groups

The chance to interact with people who fully comprehend what it's like to live with fibromyalgia is one of the biggest benefits of attending a support group. They have a distinct viewpoint and can provide insightful advice and emotional support that friends and family might not be able to provide. There is an implicit empathy and understanding among these groups that fosters a sense of belonging and togetherness.

People want to feel connected and like they belong. It might provide us great comfort to know we are not travelling alone. We can openly express ourselves in a support group without worrying about being judged because other members are also dealing with the difficulties posed by fibromyalgia. We come to grasp deeply that our challenges are real and that others have similar experiences to us through our shared stories and experiences.

Support groups develop a camaraderie that may be tremendously empowering. Seeing others overcome similar challenges with resiliency and dedication gives us strength. We draw inspiration from their triumphant stories and gain knowledge from their experiences. Even on the hardest days, we are inspired to keep moving forward by our collective triumphs. Naturally, the group dynamic facilitates the sharing of answers, coping mechanisms, and useful guidance that has worked for various people.

Support groups also offer a path for ongoing education and personal development. Patients with fibromyalgia are always looking for new strategies to control their symptoms and enhance their quality of life. We are exposed to a variety of viewpoints, approaches, and complementary and alternative medicines in these organisations. Every member contributes a different area of knowledge, be it mental health, supplementary medicine, fitness, or nutrition. By utilising this abundance of information, we can increase our comprehension and give ourselves the ability to take charge of our own health.

It's critical to keep in mind that participation in support groups involves both giving and receiving help. Sharing our personal stories and learnings makes us an inspiration to others who might be in need. Helping others through their own fibromyalgia journey helps us find recovery and gives us a sense of purpose. No matter how modest our efforts are, they have the power to significantly affect someone else's quality of life.

Beside the psychological and educational assistance, attending a support group can also positively affect our physical well-being. Studies have indicated that membership in a supportive group reduces symptoms, enhances general well-being, and increases the sense of self-efficacy that people with chronic conditions have in managing their conditions. This is partly because of the way that shared connections and the knowledge that we are not alone in our challenges reduce stress.

Stress can aggravate the symptoms of fibromyalgia, increasing pain, exhaustion, and mental discomfort. We can rely on our peers' empathy and understanding to help us deal with these stressors more skillfully if we have a support system in place. In addition, taking part in support groups may open doors to physical pursuits like walking clubs, tai chi, or moderate yoga, all of which can provide additional mental and physical comfort.

In conclusion, one of the most important choices we make on the path to wellness may be to enrol in a fibromyalgia support group. These groups provide a secure environment for connecting with people who deeply understand our struggles, offering priceless emotional support and a strong sense of belonging. We learn and develop together by exchanging knowledge and experiences, discovering fresh coping mechanisms and methods for treating our illness. Moreover, studies indicate that being a part of a support group has benefits that go beyond just improving one's emotional state, such as physical health and general well-being. We find the fortitude and resiliency required to not just endure but also flourish in the face of fibromyalgia by uniting with our peers.

Fostering Empathy and Understanding

Because its symptoms are not always apparent to others, fibromyalgia is sometimes referred to as an invisible illness. Because of this, it may be difficult for loved ones to completely comprehend and sympathise with the feelings of a person who has fibromyalgia. But with the correct resources and methods, it's possible to develop empathy and build a community that supports recovery and wellbeing for fibromyalgia sufferers and those who care about them.

Education is the first step toward developing empathy and understanding. Teaching those close to you about fibromyalgia, its symptoms, and how it affects day-to-day functioning is essential. They will be more able to comprehend the difficulties you are facing and offer you real support as a result. Start by learning as much as you can about fibromyalgia from reliable sources, including books authored by professionals in the field, credible websites, and medical publications.

After gathering this knowledge, have a conversation about fibromyalgia and its effects on your life with your loved ones. Tell them honestly and candidly about your experiences, and urge them to clarify any doubts they may have. This can help clear up any misconceptions they might have and increase empathy and understanding.

It's critical to educate those close to you about fibromyalgia, as well as the general public, in addition to yourself. This can lessen the stigma that is frequently attached to invisible illnesses and make the fibromyalgia community more accepting. Here are some tactics to think about:

1. Share your story: Individual narratives have a profound effect on people's comprehension and compassion. Take into consideration using social media, blog postings, or even local support groups to share your personal fibromyalgia experience. You may give others a better understanding of what it's like to live with this disease by sharing your storey.

2. Get involved in advocacy: Join national or local advocacy groups for fibromyalgia and take part in education efforts. This can involve planning educational activities, going to conferences, or even giving speeches in front of groups of people. In your community, you may promote understanding and good change by actively raising awareness of fibromyalgia.

3. Engage with healthcare professionals: Speak with local medical specialists and offer to discuss your fibromyalgia experiences. Hearing directly from patients can substantially improve healthcare workers' understanding and empathy towards illnesses like fibromyalgia, which are the subject of many lectures and workshops in medical schools and training programmes.

4. Utilize social media: Social media sites are excellent resources for spreading knowledge about fibromyalgia. Joining communities or groups catering to fibromyalgia may allow you to exchange materials, have discussions, and offer support to those who are also experiencing this illness. To reach more people, you might use fibromyalgia-related hashtags in your postings.

Fostering empathy and understanding also requires establishing a welcoming and inclusive workplace. This entails setting limits and telling your loved ones what you need in an efficient manner. Here are some tactics to think about:

1. Set realistic expectations: The symptoms of fibromyalgia can be unpredictable and change daily. Share this with your family and friends, and be honest with them about your limitations each day. It's critical that they comprehend that your restrictions are a function of your condition rather than a reflection of your willingness or want to engage in activities.

2. Practice open communication: Encourage open communication and give your loved ones the freedom to ask questions or voice their concerns. In a similar vein, be honest with yourself about your feelings and any routine modifications you might need to make. This can

facilitate the development of a sympathetic and perceptive dynamic in your interactions.

3. Seek support: Making use of individual treatment or joining a support group for fibromyalgia patients might help with the emotional and psychological components of the condition. While therapy can help with coping mechanisms and communication skills, sharing your experiences with like-minded folks can validate them and offer support.

4. Educate your loved ones on self-care: Not only can fibromyalgia be debilitating for those who have it, but it can also be extremely stressful for loved ones. Encourage the people you love to take care of themselves by teaching them the value of self-care. This can promote a more harmonious and encouraging atmosphere and help avoid burnout.

You can manage the difficulties of having fibromyalgia while fostering empathy and understanding in your relationships with others by putting these methods into practise. Keep in mind that developing comprehension requires patience and effort, but it is a worthwhile endeavour. By working together, we can make the world a more accepting and compassionate place for people who suffer from invisible illnesses like fibromyalgia.

Chapter 7: Enhancing Quality of Life

Pursuing Meaningful Activities

Fibromyalgia can be a debilitating and overwhelming condition that frequently traps sufferers in a vicious circle of exhaustion, pain, and diminished physical capacity. It's important to understand, though, that fibromyalgia does not sum up a person's life. Even with the limitations of this illness, each person has distinct interests, skills, and passions that can be utilised to build a meaningful existence.

Developing self-awareness is one of the keys to improving well-being and discovering meaning in the face of fibromyalgia. Importantly, in trying to cope with the day-to-day difficulties brought on by their condition, people with fibromyalgia may lose sight of who they are. Finding things to do that make you happy and fulfilled can be made easier by investigating your own interests, values, and desires. In order to truly fire their interests and give themselves a sense of purpose, I encourage my patients to engage in self-reflection, which is a crucial tool in this process.

The next step for my patients is to actively pursue their aspirations once they have developed a deeper awareness of them. Since fibromyalgia frequently impairs physical abilities and energy levels, this may be easier said than done. However, meaningful activities can be incorporated into daily life with careful planning and prioritisation. I collaborate extensively with my patients to create plans that are effective for them while taking into account their particular situation. To prevent worsening symptoms, this may entail pacing oneself, listening to one's body, and dividing activities into manageable portions.

I often advise people to investigate complementary and alternative therapies that can help manage the symptoms of fibromyalgia and enable them to participate in more fulfilling activities. By using stress-reduction and mindfulness practises, for instance, people can reduce discomfort and exhaustion and free up more energy to pursue their passions. Furthermore, self-help methods like low-impact exercise or mild stretching can improve physical capacities and facilitate participation in desired activities. I advise my patients to try different things and modify their self-care regimens in order to strike the correct balance between looking after their health and pursuing their passions.

It's also critical to understand that meaningful activities go well beyond simple pastimes or leisure activities. Making beneficial contributions to other people or the larger community can also be considered meaningful actions. One can find great joy and a sense of purpose by volunteering, performing deeds of kindness, or making a contribution to a cause that aligns with their beliefs. Engaging in this kind of activity can assist people in turning their attention from their own limits to the positive effects they can have on the lives of others. It helps people feel connected and like they belong, which is especially beneficial for fibromyalgia sufferers who frequently feel alone or misunderstood.

There may be sacrifices and adaptations needed to incorporate meaningful activities into daily life, but the benefits are priceless. Research indicates that those who participate in personally fulfilling activities have greater levels of contentment, pleasure, and general well-being. Furthermore, it has been shown that taking part in fulfilling activities lowers stress levels, enhances resilience in the face of adversity, and improves mental health. Through engaging in joyful and fulfilling activities, people with fibromyalgia can develop a stronger sense of purpose and obtain a fresh outlook on their life.

To sum up, I can't emphasise enough how important it is to pursue fulfilling hobbies as the foundation of managing fibromyalgia. These activities operate as catalysts for enjoyment, self-fulfillment, and an improved quality of life, rather than just as temporary diversion from the difficulties of the disease. People who suffer from fibromyalgia can improve their quality of life, revitalise their sense of self, and pave the way for a more fulfilling life by embracing their passions, hobbies, and purpose. I exhort my patients to look within, to find the things that really speak to them, and to let these things brighten and delight them in life. Even if fibromyalgia may have played a role in their journey, it won't define them thanks to the power of meaningful activities.

Setting Realistic Goals

As we go out on this path to become experts in managing fibromyalgia, it's critical to begin with attainable objectives. Objectives that are both realistic and customised to your particular situation. Establishing goals is essential for giving you focus, drive, and a feeling of direction while navigating the difficulties brought on by fibromyalgia. I'll go into a framework in this chapter that will assist you in setting SMART (Specific, Measurable, Achievable, Relevant, and Time-bound) objectives. I will also stress the need of setting priorities and acknowledging accomplishments in order to keep motivation high.

Let's first examine the significance of setting realistic goals before getting into the specifics of how to do so. Setting and achieving goals allows us to focus on the things that really important in life. The daily obstacles and restrictions associated with having fibromyalgia can frequently make us feel helpless and overwhelmed. We regain control and make a plan for improved health and wellbeing by setting reasonable goals.

The SMART model is among the best frameworks for creating goals. Every letter in SMART stands for a crucial component that guarantees our objectives are precise and reachable. Let's dissect it:

Specific: It's critical to be as precise as possible while establishing goals. Ideological objectives like "I want to feel better" don't offer a clear route forward. Instead, focus on one specific aspect of your life that you would like to improve and make it even more specific. For instance, "I want to increase the quality of my sleep" or "I want to lower my everyday discomfort levels."

Measurable: Progress toward an unmeasurable aim is hard to monitor. You may hold yourself accountable and evaluate the success of your tactics by setting quantifiable targets. For example, rather than just expressing, "I want to exercise more," be more specific about how many days a week you want to work out or how long each session will go.

Achievable: It's critical to establish realistic objectives. Aiming for big gains is normal, but having high expectations can only result in disappointment and annoyance. To ascertain what is practically doable for you, take into account your present situation, your constraints, and your available resources. For example, if you have never worked out before, running a marathon might not be a realistic ambition to pursue, at least not right away.

Relevant: Your goals ought to align with your beliefs and overarching objectives. Consider how reaching the objective will improve your general wellbeing. Whether your priorities are bettering your relationships, your emotional state of mind, or your physical health, it is crucial to match your goals with what matters most to you.

Time-bound: Having a deadline for your goals will help you stay motivated and focused. A deadline gives you a sense of urgency and a specific goal to strive toward. Say something like, "I want to meditate for 10 minutes every morning for the next month," as opposed to, "I want to meditate routinely."

With our structure in place, let's investigate how these SMART objectives might be used to manage fibromyalgia. Fibromyalgia can cause a variety of problems, from emotional anguish and cognitive impairment to persistent pain and exhaustion. By decomposing these difficulties into achievable objectives, we may create a comprehensive strategy for successfully controlling fibromyalgia.

Allow me to give a case study of one of my patients, Sarah, to illustrate how to use SMART goals. Three years ago, Sarah, a 35-year-old woman, received a fibromyalgia diagnosis. She frequently has excruciating pain, exhaustion, and trouble falling asleep, all of which have a negative impact on her day-to-day activities and general wellbeing. We collaborated to create SMART goals that would specifically address her needs and difficulties.

1. Specific: Sarah's main objective was to lessen her everyday suffering, which frequently reached an intolerable degree. We dissected

this objective and concentrated on methods of pain relief such heat therapy, light exercise, and meditation.

2. Measurable: Sarah kept a pain journal to record her suffering and track her progress. She may evaluate the success of her tactics and spot trends or triggers by keeping a daily log of her pain levels.

3. Achievable: Sarah's physical constraints and hectic schedule prompted us to tackle her pain management goals with a practical plan. As her tolerance increased, we began with brief meditation sessions, easy stretches, and heat therapy, progressively increasing the intensity and duration.

4. Relevant: Sarah realised that managing her pain affected not just her physical health but also her mental and emotional well-being. She understood that by better controlling her discomfort, she would have more energy and concentration to partake in her favourite hobbies.

5. Time-bound: Over the course of three months, Sarah committed to gradually increasing her daily practise of pain management strategies from 20 to 40 minutes.

Throughout this process, we have stressed the value of setting priorities and acknowledging accomplishments. Effective fibromyalgia management necessitates a multifaceted strategy that takes into account many facets of your life. You may make sure that your efforts are focused on the most crucial areas by ranking your goals according to their importance and viability.

It is also essential to recognise and honour each accomplishment of a milestone, no matter how minor. Honoring accomplishments is a potent strategy that increases drive, strengthens self-worth, and cultivates optimism. Reward yourself when you accomplish each mini-goal, whether it's lowering your pain threshold by a specific percentage or sticking to an exercise regimen for a week. These festivities act as a constant reminder of your fortitude and bolster your self-belief that you can conquer any challenge.

Recall that establishing reasonable objectives is about making progress rather than perfection. Each person's path to becoming an expert in managing their fibromyalgia is different, and the secret is to figure out what works best for you. You are creating a solid basis for a life full of energy and wellbeing by prioritising your work, creating SMART goals, and acknowledging your successes.

We will explore the importance of lifestyle alterations in the upcoming chapter, looking at how even little adjustments to our routine, nutrition, and self-care routines can make a big difference in how well we manage fibromyalgia. So come along with me as we go out on this life-changing quest to free yourself from the clutches of fibromyalgia.

Finding Joy and Fulfillment

In its most basic form, gratitude is the act of identifying and cherishing life's blessings. It is a potent tool that can assist in turning our attention from misery and anguish to the little gifts that are all around us. Gratitude is an intentional practise that opens our lives to positive energy. Gratitude can enhance our overall sense of satisfaction and boost our mental and emotional health, according to research. Gratitude can be a lifesaver when dealing with fibromyalgia, offering consolation and comfort.

Keeping a gratitude notebook is one efficient method of practising thankfulness. Spend a few minutes every day listing three things for which you are thankful. These might be as easy as a steaming cup of tea or a stunning sunset. You may teach your mind to find joy even while you are experiencing pain by keeping your attention on the good things in your life.

Techniques from positive psychology are yet another helpful tool for achieving happiness and contentment. This area of psychology is concerned with boosting happy feelings and promoting wellbeing. We can change our perspective on life and our mentality by adopting positive psychology, which will increase our level of happiness and fulfilment.

Positive affirmation practise is one well-liked positive psychology method. Positive phrases known as affirmations assist in rewiring our mental processes and beliefs. Affirmations like "I am strong and resilient" or "I have the power to conquer any difficulty" are powerful tools for self-empowerment and positive self-image reinforcement. Including affirmations in your daily practise might assist in dispelling pessimistic ideas and substituting them with empowering convictions.

Mindfulness, which is paying attention to the current moment with openness, curiosity, and without passing judgement, is another useful strategy. We can develop a sense of peace and tranquilly by engaging in mindfulness techniques like body scanning, meditation, and deep breathing. By engaging in mindfulness practises, we can better manage pain and experience joy in the here and now by developing our awareness of our bodies and emotions.

Finding happiness and contentment in life requires developing a sense of direction and significance. It provides us with a purpose for rising each morning and strengthens our will to overcome the difficulties caused by fibromyalgia. Studies have indicated that those with a strong sense of purpose in life are more likely to be happy and satisfied with their lot in life.

Examine your hobbies, values, and passions to find your purpose. What kinds of things make you happy? What problems or causes pique your interest? You may match your life to your purpose by recognising these facets of yourself, whether it is via volunteering, pursuing a creative project, or standing up for a cause that is important to you. Even in the most difficult circumstances, having purpose in your life will make you feel fulfilled and give you direction.

Apart from practising gratitude, positive psychology methods, and developing a purpose, it's critical to investigate self-care activities that enhance your mental, emotional, and physical health. Frequent symptoms of fibromyalgia include fatigue, muscle soreness, and irregular sleep patterns. Taking part in activities that encourage self-care and relaxation can help reduce these symptoms and improve your general quality of life.

Try out various self-care methods, such as massage therapy, aromatherapy, light exercise, or taking up enjoyable hobbies. Make rest a priority and make sure you receive adequate sleep every night. Fill your body with wholesome nutrients that will boost your vitality and improve your overall health. By looking after your whole self, you lay the groundwork for achieving happiness and contentment in your life.

To sum up, although fibromyalgia might bring about a lot of difficulties, it doesn't define you or your capacity for happiness and contentment. You can traverse the nuances of this condition and discover a vast amount of joy and fulfilment by practising gratitude, positive psychology skills, and developing a feeling of purpose and meaning. Always keep in mind that you are the writer of your own life, and using these techniques will enable you to create a happy, resilient, and personally fulfilling storey. Accept the path and give yourself permission to grow in spite of the obstacles.

Embracing Self-Care and Self-Compassion

Routines for self-care are essential to controlling the symptoms of fibromyalgia and enhancing general wellbeing. These practises entail making conscious decisions to support one's mental, emotional, and physical well-being. As a physician and health and wellness coach, I have personally witnessed the significant impact that integrating self-care habits can have on my patients' lives. People with fibromyalgia can benefit from decreased pain, better sleep, more energy, and improved mood by adding self-care rituals into their daily routines.

A self-care practise that people with fibromyalgia can follow is making sleep and rest a priority. People with fibromyalgia frequently find it difficult to get restorative sleep because of their pain and suffering. On the other hand, people can enhance the quality of their sleep by establishing a calming nighttime routine that includes activities like reading a book, having a warm bath, or meditating. Better sleep patterns can also be attained by maintaining a regular sleep regimen and furnishing a cosy sleeping space.

Light exercise and mobility is another self-care practise that helps help people with fibromyalgia. Numerous advantages of exercise for fibromyalgia sufferers have been demonstrated, including pain reduction, mood enhancement, and general physical strength enhancement. But it's important to pick low-impact activities that don't make your symptoms worse. Exercises like yoga, tai chi, swimming, and walking can help to maintain flexibility and strength while being easy on the joints and muscles.

A powerful discipline that many with fibromyalgia neglect is self-acceptance. It entails accepting and embracing oneself together with all of the mental and physical difficulties that the illness presents. Flare-ups can happen at any time with fibromyalgia, which can be surprising and frustrating. But through practising self-acceptance, people can let go of their judgement of themselves and accept their journey with empathy and understanding. Through self-improvement and resilience building, this practise helps people deal gracefully with the ups and downs of living with fibromyalgia.

For people with fibromyalgia, self-advocacy is just as important as self-acceptance in improving their quality of life. Actively engaging in healthcare decisions, expressing needs and concerns to medical experts, and enlisting the aid of others are all components of self-advocacy. It guarantees that people's opinions are heard in the healthcare system and gives them the power to take control of their health and well-being. People can work more productively with their healthcare providers to create individualised treatment plans and obtain the resources they need by learning about fibromyalgia and its management.

It is impossible to overestimate the significance of self-compassion and self-care in the efficient management of fibromyalgia. Studies have indicated that engaging in self-care and self-compassion practises can yield favourable outcomes for pain perception, stress levels, and emotional health. Self-care routines enable people to nourish their bodies and brains, lowering stress and fostering calm. Comparably, cultivating self-compassion entails being kind, patient, and understanding to oneself, all of which have a positive effect on one's mental and emotional health.

Moreover, coping mechanisms and self-compassion and self-care are intimately related. People with fibromyalgia symptoms need to learn good coping mechanisms for pain, exhaustion, and other difficulties. People can proactively address these symptoms and lessen their influence on day-to-day living by adopting self-care techniques. Furthermore, self-compassion gives people the emotional support they need to deal with the psychological and physical difficulties brought on by fibromyalgia. By enabling people to acknowledge and give meaning to their experiences, it promotes self-determination and fortitude.

In summary, adopting self-care and self-compassion is essential for fibromyalgia sufferers to improve their quality of life. Through implementing self-care routines, engaging in self-advocacy, and practising self-acceptance, people can enhance their general well-being and effectively manage their symptoms. Self-care practises can reduce discomfort, enhance the quality of sleep, and increase vitality. Examples of these practises include making rest and sleep a priority and doing light exercise. People who are self-advocate and self-acceptant are better able to deal with the difficulties of having fibromyalgia with fortitude and grace. People can develop a loving and understanding relationship with themselves and improve their mental and emotional health by engaging in self-compassion practises. In the end, fibromyalgia sufferers can enjoy happy lives and take charge of their health and wellbeing by practising self-care and self-compassion.

Chapter 8: Overcoming Challenges and Flare-ups

Understanding Flare-ups

Fibromyalgia is a long-term medical disorder that is typified by a variety of symptoms, including exhaustion and extensive pain. However, precisely what are flare-ups? A flare-up is essentially a period of time during which symptoms worsen and escalate. These episodes can significantly affect day-to-day living and extend for a few days to many weeks.

The presence of triggers is essential to the occurrence of flare-ups. Although the precise triggers can differ from person to person, fibromyalgia sufferers often experience exacerbation of symptoms due to several common circumstances. One of the main things that sets off flare-ups is stress. Stress hormones like cortisol are released by the body in response to physical, mental, or psychological stress, and they have the potential to intensify pain signals and symptoms.

Overdoing things is another typical trigger. A flare-up may result from pushing ourselves too hard, either mentally or physically. Striking the correct balance between work and relaxation is crucial to avoid pushing ourselves too far and possibly setting off a flare-up.

Weather variations can also affect the symptoms of fibromyalgia. For example, a lot of people with fibromyalgia claim that chilly weather exacerbates their pain and stiffness. The first step to successfully controlling flare-ups is realising these triggers and developing the ability to recognise them in our own life.

It's critical to recognise the signs of a flare-up. In addition to the persistent pain and exhaustion that people with fibromyalgia endure, flare-ups can cause a variety of other symptoms. Increased sensitivity to pressure and touch, sleep difficulties, anxiety, melancholy, headaches, gastrointestinal problems, and cognitive impairments commonly referred to as "fibro fog" are a few of these. When these symptoms flare up, we may feel overwhelmed and unable to function normally due to their intensity.

A flare-length up's can differ significantly from person to person. Shorter, more frequent flare-ups may occur for some people, whereas lengthier exacerbation periods interspersed with remission periods may occur for others. We can better prepare for and handle our own flare-ups if we are aware of our own habits.

Proactive management and reduction of flare-up frequency and intensity are necessary. It is imperative to devise tactics that tackle the physiological and psychological dimensions of fibromyalgia. Changes in lifestyle are essential. This entails keeping a consistent sleep pattern, doing physical therapy or mild exercise, and implementing a nutritious diet that stays away from trigger foods like processed sweets and coffee.

Techniques from psychology and counselling may also be helpful in controlling flare-ups. For example, cognitive-behavioral therapy (CBT) can assist people in reframing unfavourable ideas and creating coping strategies for handling stress and suffering. Deep breathing exercises, meditation, and relaxation techniques are examples of mind-body therapies that can help reduce the symptoms of a flare-up.

Self-help methods are essential weapons in the armoury for preventing flare-ups. This entails setting aside time for self-care and pacing oneself while juggling work and relaxation. It's critical to pay attention to our body during flare-ups and allow ourselves the space and time we require to heal.

Lastly, managing flare-ups can also greatly benefit from complementary and alternative therapies. For those with fibromyalgia, methods such as massage therapy, acupuncture, and herbal therapies have demonstrated promise in lowering pain and enhancing general wellbeing. It's crucial to investigate these choices after speaking with medical experts who specialise in fibromyalgia.

In summary, comprehension of the nature of fibromyalgia flare-ups is essential for efficient management and a decrease in both frequency and severity. We can learn to manage flare-ups more easily and enhance our overall quality of life by identifying triggers, recognising symptoms, and creating a comprehensive plan that includes lifestyle modifications, counselling and psychology-related techniques, self-help strategies, and complementary and alternative therapies.

Developing Coping Strategies

Reduction strategies are essential for treating flare-ups of fibromyalgia. Both the body and the mind can be negatively impacted by chronic pain and exhaustion, which can exacerbate symptoms and lead to stress. People can improve their general well-being and obtain much-needed relief by practising relaxation techniques.

Deep breathing is one of the most well-known methods of relaxing. Taking slow, deep breaths helps the body release tension and foster calmness. It's a simple yet effective technique. Shut your eyes, take a deep breath through your nose, hold it for a short while, and then gently release the breath through your mouth. Several times over, repeat this procedure while paying attention to how your breath feels entering and leaving your body. Imagine the stress dissipating with each breath, to be replaced with a profound sense of peace.

Progressive muscular relaxation, when combined with deep breathing, can be an effective strategy for controlling flare-ups. This method, which helps release tension in the body and mind, entails methodically tensing and relaxing various muscle groups. Start by concentrating on one particular muscle group, like your shoulders. Your shoulder muscles should be tense. Hold the position for a short while, then relax. After letting the tension leave your body, proceed to the next muscle group and repeat the technique until your entire body is relaxed. Progressive muscle relaxation is a handy coping mechanism for fibromyalgia flare-ups because it can be used in the comfort of your own home.

For people with fibromyalgia, pain management approaches are just as important as relaxing techniques. One of the main symptoms of this illness is chronic pain, which can be significantly improved by finding efficient pain relief techniques.

Heat treatment is one pain management technique that has showed promise. In addition to improving blood flow and relaxing muscles, applying heat to sore spots can temporarily reduce discomfort. Heating pads, warm baths, and hot packs can all help with this. Try a variety of techniques to see which one suits you the best, and make heat treatment a regular part of your day to help you effectively manage your pain.

Gentle exercise is another important pain management technique that shouldn't be disregarded. Even though it might seem strange to move when in pain, light exercise can really assist lower pain levels and enhance general function. Walking, swimming, and yoga are examples of low-impact workouts that can help build muscle, improve flexibility, and produce endorphins, the body's natural painkillers. Start out softly and work your way up to a higher intensity and longer workout time. Always pay attention to your body's needs and modify your workout regimen to fit your unique capabilities.

Creating emotional resilience is a crucial part of creating coping mechanisms for managing fibromyalgia. It can be difficult to manage a chronic illness on a physical and emotional level. To overcome obstacles and preserve wellbeing, it's critical to cultivate resilience and an optimistic outlook.

Cognitive behavioural therapy is one method that can assist in fostering emotional resilience (CBT). The goal of CBT is to recognise and alter harmful thinking processes and behaviour patterns that fuel emotional suffering. People can cultivate a more resilient mindset and more effectively manage the difficulties associated with fibromyalgia by confronting negative thoughts and substituting them with more realistic and upbeat ones. Gaining knowledge of and practising these approaches in your everyday life can be greatly aided by working with a licenced CBT therapist or counsellor.

Self-care is a crucial element of emotional resiliency. Taking good care of oneself is essential for treating fibromyalgia, both mentally and physically. This can involve things like taking up a hobby, spending time with loved ones, practising mindfulness and meditation, and making rest and relaxation a priority. People with fibromyalgia who prioritise self-care are better able to manage the ups and downs of their condition and develop emotional resilience.

In conclusion, it is critical for people with fibromyalgia to learn coping mechanisms in order to handle flare-ups and overcome obstacles. People can overcome obstacles and prosper in the face of hardship by implementing pain management tactics, emotional resilience skills, and relaxation techniques into their daily routine. Always keep in mind that you should customise these coping mechanisms to fit your own requirements and preferences by determining what works best for you. You are capable of living a more contented and balanced life if you are persistent and take an active approach to treating your fibromyalgia.

Seeking Support During Difficult Times

Family and close friends are examples of loved ones who can provide unwavering support throughout trying times. They are there to help us through the highs and lows of living with fibromyalgia by providing love, support, and encouragement. They frequently serve as a sounding board for us, enabling us to voice our worries and concerns without fear of repercussions. Their compassion and empathy can be consoling because they serve as a reminder that we are not alone in our troubles.

Family members can offer helpful advice as well as emotional support. They can assist with everyday chores like cleaning or food shopping, which can become too much to do when fibromyalgia flares up. They can also go with us to doctor's appointments, acting as a second pair of ears and aiding in our memory of crucial details. The worry and anxiety that frequently accompany medical appointments can be reduced when we have someone by our sides.

As vital as family members are in our network of support, medical experts too have a key position. As a medical professional, I know how crucial it is to choose a skilled and sympathetic healthcare practitioner. A fibromyalgia specialist in the medical field can offer important advice and insight into treating the illness.

Healthcare providers can evaluate our symptoms, track our development, and provide individualised treatment plans throughout appointments. They can provide advice on lifestyle changes that can help reduce symptoms, like regular exercise, good sleep hygiene, and nutritional changes. Depending on how severe our symptoms are, they might also recommend medication or other therapies.

Healthcare practitioners can offer emotional support and validation in addition to their medical competence. They are sympathetic to our experiences and are aware of the difficulties that fibromyalgia sufferers have. They can cheer and reassure us, serving as a reminder that our illness does not define who we are.

Another helpful tool in our fibromyalgia journey is a support group. These groups bring together people who, because they are facing similar difficulties, have firsthand knowledge of our struggles. They offer a secure and encouraging space for us to talk about our struggles, worries, and victories.

Being a part of a support group might make us feel more understood and less alone. It provides a chance to pick up new skills, see the world from other angles, and find coping mechanisms that have worked for other participants. Additionally, support groups may invite specialists or guest speakers to provide additional information about managing fibromyalgia and self-care practises.

Support groups can provide a forum for helpful advice in addition to emotional support. Members may exchange resources, including doctors, therapists, and complementary therapies that they have found effective. They can provide guidance on financial aid options, insurance policies, and navigating the healthcare system. In order to fully understand fibromyalgia, a support group's combined expertise and experience might be quite helpful.

In conclusion, getting help when things get tough is crucial for managing fibromyalgia. Support groups, medical professionals, and loved ones all have special roles to play in offering direction, compassion, and useful help. Their presence in our life gives us a sense of empowerment, understanding, and support as we deal with the difficulties caused by fibromyalgia.

I urge you to build and tend to your support network as we set out on this journey. See a doctor who specialises in treating fibromyalgia, enlist in a support group, and rely on your loved ones for both practical and emotional help. Recall that there are people and tools available to assist you in achieving full management of your fibromyalgia. You are not alone. If we work together, we can overcome this illness and prosper.

Maintaining Resilience and Optimism

Let's start by examining the effectiveness of positive thinking. Positive thinking is a strong tool that can change your perspective and give you the confidence to take on obstacles head-on. It's not just a catchphrase or slogan. Negative ideas can quickly take control of your mind when dealing with chronic pain and the challenges that come with it, sending you into a depressing downward spiral. Still, you may rewire your brain to develop a more positive attitude on life by making a conscious decision to concentrate on positive thoughts.

A useful method for promoting optimistic thinking is the daily affirmation exercise. Repetition of empowering affirmations, either mentally or out loud, usually in front of a mirror, serves as a means of reinforcing positive self-perception and self-worth. By including affirmations in your daily routine, you are telling yourself that you are strong and resilient and that you can conquer any obstacles that fibromyalgia may provide.

Reframing failures is another way to stay resilient and optimistic. Experiencing setbacks or hurdles can naturally lead to feelings of discouragement and failure. But you may turn these failures into stepping stones to success if you reframe them as chances for learning and development. Consider setbacks as important lessons that might help you move forward in your quest for optimal fibromyalgia management rather than as failures.

Journaling is one method that can help with rephrasing failures. Every day, set aside some time to consider the difficulties you've encountered and the knowledge you've gained. Once you've written down any negative feelings or thoughts, try to rephrase them in a way that feels more empowering and uplifting. For instance, reframe a very painful flare-up as a chance to rest and recharge so that your body can repair and regenerate, rather than seeing it as a setback.

Remaining resilient and optimistic requires not just thinking positively but also rephrasing failures and developing a growth mentality. The idea that one's skills and intelligence may be enhanced via commitment and effort is known as a growth mindset. With fibromyalgia's chronic pain and limitations, it's simple to get stuck in your ways and think there's not much you can do to get better. On the other hand, you expose yourself to countless opportunities and growth potential when you adopt a growth mentality.

Gratitude is a habit that helps cultivate a growth mentality. Every day, set aside some time to consider all of the blessings in your life, no matter how minor they may appear. By focusing on the positive aspects of your life rather than the challenges posed by fibromyalgia, you can cultivate thankfulness and become more resilient and upbeat. You may keep a mindset that supports progress and personal development by appreciating the little things in life.

Additionally, getting help from those who are aware of your difficulties can go a long way toward preserving your optimism and resilience. A sense of community and priceless emotional support can be obtained by attending support meetings or going to counselling. Being surrounded by people who have conquered comparable obstacles might provide as inspiration and motivation for you as you navigate your own fibromyalgia management journey.

Finally, it's critical to put self-care first and partake in pursuits that make you happy and fulfilled. Taking good care of your mental, emotional, and physical health can make you more resilient and upbeat. Take up hobbies, yoga, nature walks, or other pleasurable and relaxing activities that you enjoy to help you decompress. You are providing yourself with the fortitude and resiliency required to handle the difficulties presented by fibromyalgia by taking care of your mind, body, and spirit.

In summary, preserving optimism and resilience is critical to treating fibromyalgia well. Through the application of positive thinking, repositioning obstacles, developing a growth mentality, getting help, and making self-care a priority, you can effectively manage the difficulties associated with fibromyalgia and eventually achieve mastery. Never forget that you are strong enough to design a life that is not limited by your fibromyalgia but rather strengthened by your inner fortitude and optimism.

Chapter 9: Empowering Self-Advocacy

Effective Communication With Healthcare Providers

It's critical to understand that medical professionals are not mind readers. Though we are specialists in our domains, we are dependent on our patients' candid and open communication in order to completely comprehend their requirements and worries. Since fibromyalgia is a complicated and multifaceted disorder, it is even more important to communicate effectively in order to make sure that patients receive the specialised care that they need.

Posing questions is a crucial component of good communication. Patients are better able to comprehend their disease and available treatments as a result. Make sure you have a list of questions ready for your medical appointment. This guarantees that during the session, you won't overlook any crucial details. As questions come up, it can be useful to jot them down so you have them for later.

Some examples of questions you may want to ask your healthcare provider include:

1. What are the potential causes or triggers of my fibromyalgia symptoms?

2. What are the treatment options available to me?

3. What are the potential side effects of the medications you are recommending?

4. How long will it take for the treatment to show results?

5. Are there any complementary therapies or lifestyle modifications that may benefit me?

6. How can I manage my symptoms on a day-to-day basis?

Recall that asking questions is not an indication of ignorance or weakness. It indicates that you are committed to determining the best course of action for yourself and that you are willing to play an active role in your healthcare.

A crucial component of good communication is voicing concerns. It is important that you discuss any concerns or questions you may have with your healthcare provider regarding your treatment plan. Only once they are aware of your problems will they be able to solve them. It's okay to voice your opinions, even if they don't seem important. Your medical professional is available to listen to you and guide you on your path to improved health.

Making decisions about healthcare requires active engagement. In your treatment plan, you ought to constantly feel like an equal participant. This entails participating in the decision-making process and making your opinion known. Recall that you are in charge of your body, and that your healthcare practitioner is there to support, encourage, and provide you the tools you need to manage the symptoms of your fibromyalgia.

To actively participate in your healthcare decisions, you can:

1. Educate yourself: Find out more about alternative therapies, fibromyalgia, and available treatments. You may make more assured decisions regarding your health if you are knowledgeable.

2. Keep a symptom journal: Keep a record of your symptoms, triggers, and response to therapy. This can aid in decision-making and give your healthcare provider insightful information.

3. Seek second opinions: Getting a second opinion is totally fine if you are unsure about your diagnosis or current course of therapy. This can bring you a fresh viewpoint and assist you in making better health-related decisions.

4. Trust your instincts: Your body knows you best. Trust your gut and let your healthcare practitioner know if something about your treatment plan doesn't feel right or if you have any doubts.

Active listening is another essential component of effective communication. It's critical that you pay close attention to the counsel, suggestions, and clarifications provided by your healthcare provider. If something is unclear to you, don't be afraid to ask for clarification or to take notes. By attentively listening, you can make sure that any decisions you make are supported by correct information and that you completely understand your treatment alternatives.

To sum up, good communication between patients and medical professionals is essential for controlling fibromyalgia. Important elements of this process include voicing concerns, asking questions, and actively engaging in healthcare decisions. Recall that your voice counts and that you are an essential component of your own healthcare team. You can make sure you get the greatest fibromyalgia care and treatment by becoming an active member of your healthcare provider's team.

Navigating Healthcare Systems

I am a fibromyalgia specialist medical doctor and health and wellness coach, so I am aware of the difficulties people encounter when attempting to make their way through the healthcare system. Although the system can be daunting and perplexing, you can make sure you get the assistance and care you require by arming yourself with the appropriate information and coping mechanisms.

Knowing what is covered by your health insurance is the first step towards navigating the healthcare system. It is imperative that you go over your insurance coverage and become acquainted with the particular benefits and restrictions associated with fibromyalgia. This will assist you in comprehending the therapies and drugs that are covered, along with any referral or authorization criteria that may be required. Please do not hesitate to contact your insurance provider for clarification if you have any questions or concerns regarding your coverage.

The next stage is to compile and arrange your medical records after you have a firm grasp of your insurance coverage. This contains your fibromyalgia-related test findings, treatment plans, and medication history. You can ensure that you receive the right care and that you communicate with healthcare providers more effectively if you have this information at your fingertips. To carry your medical records to appointments, you can organise them into a digital folder or binder.

It's crucial to know how to properly convey your wants to healthcare providers in addition to keeping your medical records organised. Locate a primary care physician who is either willing to learn about fibromyalgia or is educated about it. This will be your primary point of contact for scheduling appointments with specialists and managing your overall treatment. It's okay to get a second opinion or look for a specialist who specialises in treating fibromyalgia if your current primary care physician does not understand fibromyalgia.

Bring a list of questions and concerns with you when you visit a healthcare physician. This will make it more likely that your needs will be met in the course of the appointment. Jot down any symptoms you are having, any changes to your health, and any previous treatments you have taken. With this information, your healthcare professional will be able to design a treatment plan specifically for you and gain a thorough insight of your fibromyalgia experience.

To properly treat your fibromyalgia symptoms, you might need to see a number of specialists in addition to your main care physician. Rheumatologists, neurologists, and pain management experts are a few examples of these professionals. It's critical to look for healthcare professionals with experience managing chronic pain problems like fibromyalgia. Your health care physician may be able to recommend someone, or you may look for local experts who specialise in treating fibromyalgia.

Making appointments is the next step after you have determined which specialists are best for your needs. It is imperative that you take charge of your healthcare and don't wait for appointments to be made for you. Keep in mind that meetings with specialists should be scheduled as soon as possible because they can have lengthy wait times. To ensure that you don't miss any appointments, make sure to create reminders and keep track of all the dates and hours of your appointments.

To effectively manage fibromyalgia, it's critical to have access to the right resources and support in addition to specialised care. This can include educational materials, internet discussion boards, and support groups. Making connections with other fibromyalgia sufferers can offer a platform for advice and coping technique sharing, as well as a sense of validation and empathy. Furthermore, gaining knowledge about fibromyalgia from reliable sources can enable you to speak out for yourself more effectively and make wise healthcare decisions.

Finally, it is imperative that you actively participate in your own healthcare management. This entails sticking to prescribed course of action, routinely checking in with medical professionals, and speaking up for oneself when needed. To keep track of your symptoms, medical interventions, and any changes to your condition, keep a journal. Not only may this data assist you in tracking your development, but it also offers insightful information that you can discuss with your medical team.

It might be intimidating to navigate the complicated healthcare systems, but you can make sure you get the best care possible for your fibromyalgia by following a step-by-step plan and getting the support you need. You are advocating for yourself and enhancing your quality of life by being aware of your health insurance coverage, keeping your medical records organised, and making sure that healthcare providers know what you need. Recall that you have resources and experts at your disposal to assist you at every turn on this trip; you are not alone.

Advocating for Your Needs and Rights

1. Understanding the Importance of Self-Advocacy:

It is imperative to acknowledge the significance of self-advocacy first and foremost. Patients with fibromyalgia encounter particular difficulties that call for initiative. We can make sure that our healthcare providers are aware of our unique demands and adjust our treatment plans by advocating for ourselves. Additionally, self-advocacy gives us the ability to take charge of our own health and wellbeing by enabling us to seek the treatment we need and make educated decisions.

2. Developing Assertiveness Skills:

Being forceful is a key component of self-advocacy. Being assertive entails confidently and respectfully stating our demands and desires. It's critical to keep in mind that we have the right to have our concerns acknowledged and to be heard. Acquiring assertiveness skills can be immensely liberating, and it's a tool that we can use in many areas of our lives, not just medical situations.

It can be beneficial to practise assertive communication tactics in order to build assertiveness skills. Use "I" phrases, for instance, to convey your needs and worries to your healthcare professional while you're talking about your symptoms or treatment alternatives. Try expressing, "I feel angry when my issues aren't taken seriously," rather than, "You never listen to me." Using this method makes it easier to communicate your thoughts and feelings without criticising the other person. Setting limits and saying no when it's necessary are other aspects of being assertive. Recall that your body and experiences are your domain of expertise.

3. Seeking Second Opinions:

Having the capacity to seek second perspectives is another crucial component of self-advocacy. This is especially crucial if you are in the process of making treatment decisions or if you believe your present healthcare provider is not giving enough attention to your concerns.

Getting a second opinion can bring you new insight and reveal therapeutic possibilities you had not previously thought of.

Getting all of your test results and medical documents together to give to your new healthcare professional might be beneficial when getting a second opinion. By doing this, you can be sure they have all the data they need to evaluate your situation intelligently. Recall that it is your responsibility as a patient to look for the best care available to you.

4. Accessing Disability Accommodations:

Fibromyalgia can be a crippling illness that makes it difficult for us to work or do daily chores. In certain instances, obtaining accommodations for disabilities could be essential to guarantee our continued full participation in society. This can entail requesting disability benefits if you are unable to work or making adaptations to your workspace or schedule as part of workplace accommodations.

It can be difficult to obtain accommodations for people with disabilities, but it's crucial to keep trying. Begin by learning about the rules and legislation pertaining to accommodations for people with disabilities in your nation or area. Learn about your rights and the precise actions you must take in order to receive these accommodations. Contacting organisations or support groups that specialise in standing up for people with fibromyalgia or other chronic ailments may also be beneficial.

Recall that standing up for your demands and rights may call for endurance and tolerance. Even while not everyone can relate to or validate your experiences, you shouldn't let that stop you from standing up and demanding what is rightfully yours. Assemble a strong support system of family, friends, and professionals who can mentor and encourage you on this journey.

In summary, your quality of life and general well-being depend on you as a patient with fibromyalgia speaking up for your needs and rights. You may make sure that your voice is heard and that your concerns are taken seriously by getting second views, practising assertiveness, and requesting modifications for people with disabilities. Never forget that you are not travelling alone. When we work together, we can make a world where people with fibromyalgia are respected and cared for.

Building a Supportive Healthcare Team

It is essential to have a healthcare team that is aware of the particular difficulties and complications associated with managing fibromyalgia. As they say, "It takes a village," and when it comes to your health, this is really true. Having worked for many years as a medical practitioner and health and wellness coach, I have witnessed firsthand the positive impact that a caring healthcare team can have on fibromyalgia patients' lives.

Your primary care physician is the cornerstone of your healthcare team. The cornerstone of your medical care is your primary care physician, who will also be instrumental in organising the entirety of your treatment regimen. They will serve as your primary contact for routine screenings, check-ups, and general health issues. Locating a primary care physician who understands fibromyalgia and is prepared to collaborate closely with you to treat your symptoms is crucial. They will act as your champion and gatekeeper when it comes to obtaining more medical care, and they will frequently refer you to other specialists when necessary.

In addition to your main care physician, you might find it helpful to speak with a variety of experts who specialise in different aspects of managing fibromyalgia. These experts may include, among others, neurologists, psychologists, rheumatologists, and pain management specialists. For example, a rheumatologist can assist in diagnosing and treating musculoskeletal diseases and can also assist in evaluating and treating fibromyalgia symptoms. Pain management specialists are knowledgeable about various pain management techniques and can assist you in obtaining relief from the persistent pain linked to fibromyalgia. Neurologists can help identify and treat any problems with the neurological system that might be causing your symptoms. Finally, a psychologist can offer you coping mechanisms to improve your general well-being and assist you in navigating the psychological and emotional components of having fibromyalgia.

Although these experts are essential in treating particular facets of fibromyalgia, it's crucial to keep in mind that the illness is complicated and necessitates a multimodal approach to care. This is where the role of allied health professionals is needed. These experts, who focus on complementary and alternative therapies, offer a priceless addition to standard medical care.

A registered dietician, sometimes known as a nutritionist, is one type of allied healthcare worker. Together, you may develop a personalised food plan that promotes your general health and wellbeing. They can assist you in addressing any vitamin deficiencies and optimising your nutrition to reduce symptoms through dietary alterations. For instance, some foods have anti-inflammatory qualities that may help lessen pain and discomfort, while others may cause inflammation and aggravate the symptoms of fibromyalgia. A nutritionist can also help you make better eating choices, which will improve your general quality of life and energy levels.

Physical therapists are another allied health professional that is worthwhile to take into account. They can help you become more flexible and strong overall, as well as enhance your ability to perform physically and reduce pain. A physical therapist can design a customised training regimen that takes into consideration your unique requirements and constraints. They can aid in pain alleviation and mobility improvement by combining methods including manual therapy, stretching exercises, and low-impact aerobic workouts. Moreover, physical therapy can help with fatigue reduction and better sleep patterns, two issues that fibromyalgia sufferers frequently face.

Seeking assistance from practitioners of complementary and alternative medicine can be beneficial in addition to these doctors. This could involve extra options for pain management and general well-being, such as massage therapists, acupuncturists, and chiropractors. Numerous fibromyalgia sufferers report experiencing notable symptom relief with these techniques, while individual results may vary in their usefulness. However, it's crucial to speak with your primary care physician and make sure that any alternative treatments you choose are suitable and safe for your particular situation.

Finally, we must not undervalue the role that mental health plays in the overall care of fibromyalgia. It is imperative to seek the guidance of a mental health expert due to the significant influence that chronic pain and other symptoms have on mental well-being. Psychologists, therapists, and counsellors can offer you a safe place to talk about your worries as well as coping skills training and assistance in navigating the emotional difficulties of having fibromyalgia. They can help you deal with any anxiety, depression, or other mental health issues that may surface as a result of your disease and can also support you in creating good coping methods.

Establishing an encouraging healthcare team is a continuous effort that calls for trust, cooperation, and open communication. By collaborating with your team of medical specialists, you may develop a comprehensive treatment plan that takes into account every aspect of living with fibromyalgia. This strategy makes sure you get the all-encompassing care you require to successfully control your symptoms and enhance your general quality of life.

To sum up, developing a caring healthcare team is crucial for managing fibromyalgia effectively. As the cornerstone of your healthcare team, your primary care physician collaborates with specialists and other medical experts to deliver all-encompassing care. They will work together to create a treatment plan that takes into account the psychological, emotional, and physical elements of fibromyalgia and makes sure you get the help you need along the way. Recall that you don't have to deal with fibromyalgia alone; you can take charge of your health and start along the path to optimal well-being with a supportive healthcare team by your side.

Chapter 10: Thriving With Fibromyalgia

Stories of Resilience and Triumph

I'd like to start by telling the tale of Sarah, a 45-year-old lady who was identified as having fibromyalgia in her early 20s. Sarah was horrified to learn of her news at first. She believed that her life was ended and that she would never be able to lead the fulfilling life she had dreamed of. But Sarah is a fighter, and she chose to take charge of her health rather than give up.

Sarah committed to controlling her symptoms and enhancing her general health. She started by implementing major lifestyle adjustments, such as starting an exercise programme and eating a nutritious diet. She began doing yoga and meditation, which assisted her in controlling her discomfort and lowering her stress levels. Sarah also sought assistance from other medical specialists, such as psychologists, dietitians, and physical therapists, who assisted her in creating coping mechanisms and keeping an optimistic outlook.

Sarah's tenacity and dedication paid off over time. She not only controlled her symptoms but also had a fruitful and prosperous writing career. Sarah now serves as an encouragement to other fibromyalgia sufferers. She frequently gives talks at conferences and support groups, and she also writes a blog where she shares her experiences and management techniques for the illness. Sarah's tale is a living example of the strength of perseverance and the capacity to overcome hardship.

Another amazing tale of perseverance comes from Mark, a 38-year-old man who for years had been suffering from severe pain and weariness before receiving a fibromyalgia diagnosis. Due to his illness, Mark found it challenging to maintain a consistent work schedule or take part in his favourite pastimes. Because so many people around him questioned the veracity of his ailment, he felt alone and misunderstood.

But Mark didn't want his fibromyalgia to define who he was. He made it his mission to become as knowledgeable as he could about the illness and its treatment options. He tried a range of therapies, such as lifestyle modifications, complementary therapies, and medicine. Mark eventually discovered a mix of medications that were effective for him after years of trial and error.

But Mark's adventure didn't end there. His goal was to help others going through similar struggles by using his experiences. He founded a nonprofit organisation to assist those who are affected by fibromyalgia and turned into an advocate for raising awareness of the ailment. Mark provides financial aid for treatment alternatives, support groups, and instructional materials through his foundation. He is a brilliant illustration of fortitude and success in the face of difficulty.

Finally, I'd want to tell the tale of Emily, a 32-year-old who was identified as having fibromyalgia at an early age. Emily didn't allow her illness stop her from reaching her goals, though. She decided to become a doctor and rose to prominence as a major authority on fibromyalgia. Emily's dual viewpoint as a patient and a medical practitioner enabled her to significantly advance the discipline.

Emily's research yielded novel therapeutic approaches and strategies for enhancing the quality of life for fibromyalgia sufferers. Through the integrative approach she established, patients can now address both the physical and emotional components of their ailment, as traditional medicine is combined with holistic therapies. In addition to helping numerous people find comfort, Emily's effort has raised fibromyalgia's profile in the medical community and improved knowledge of the condition.

These are only a handful of the numerous people who have overcome the difficulties caused by fibromyalgia. There are many more. Though every person's journey is different, they are all united by a shared spirit of will, fortitude, and optimism. By telling you these tales, I want to encourage and inspire you to think that you are capable of overcoming fibromyalgia's obstacles and leading a happy life. Never forget that there is always hope for a better future and that you are not alone on this road.

Finding Purpose and Meaning

I was first witness to the personal toll that fibromyalgia can have on people when I started my career as a medical doctor with a focus on managing this ailment. I saw firsthand the physical suffering, mental anguish, and hopelessness that frequently followed the diagnosis. I realised that treating my patients' emotional and psychological needs was just as important as treating their physical problems if I wanted to genuinely help them thrive.

Throughout the years of my work, I have found that one of the most important aspects of managing fibromyalgia is having meaning and purpose in life. Treating the symptoms is not enough; we also need to work toward making life worthwhile. Finding one's hobbies and interests—those pursuits that provide happiness, contentment, and a feeling of direction—is the first step in doing this.

To begin this process, set aside some time for introspection. Knowing what really matters to you and who you are at your heart is vital. This could entail analysing your values, evaluating your talents and shortcomings, and figuring out what kinds of things and experiences really speak to you.

It's time to investigate your passions after you have a better understanding of who you are. What piques your curiosity? What pursuits make you happy and fulfilled? This might be as easy as writing, drawing, gardening, or volunteering. Finding something that piques your interest and gives you a sense of aliveness and connection to the outside world is crucial.

Now that you know what your passions are, it's time to engage in fulfilling activities. This could entail making a plan, acting, and establishing objectives. It's crucial to keep in mind that discovering meaning and purpose may not always be simple. There can be difficulties, roadblocks, and difficulties in the path. These difficulties, meanwhile, might also present chances for development and education.

It's critical to treat oneself with kindness when dealing with fibromyalgia and to approach your goals patiently and mindfully. Respect your body's limits and pay attention to it. Take it slow and strike a balance between honouring your body's need for rest and recuperation and pushing yourself to improve.

Developing a sense of contentment involves more than merely engaging in enjoyable activities. It also entails fostering connections, interacting with people, and giving back to a cause greater than oneself. This could entail creating a network of friends and family that are sympathetic to your situation and understand your journey. It could also entail volunteering or performing deeds of service to the community.

It's critical to keep in mind that each person's journey toward meaning and purpose is distinct. What makes one person happy and fulfilled might not be meaningful to another. Respecting your own path and restraining yourself from comparing yourself to others are essential. Accept who you are and listen to your own inner guidance system.

It could be beneficial to ask for advice and encouragement from those who have been through a similar situation along the way. As you travel your own path towards meaning and purpose, joining support groups, going to conferences or workshops, or getting advice from a health and wellness coach can all offer insightful information and assistance.

Recall that discovering meaning and purpose in life is a lifetime journey rather than a destination. Your hobbies and passions may vary as circumstances and life change. Accept that life is fluid and have an open mind to new possibilities and experiences. You will keep building a life that is defined by the meaning and purpose you give to it, not by fibromyalgia, with every step you take forward.

To sum up, discovering meaning and purpose in life is crucial to effective fibromyalgia treatment. Merely treating the condition's physical symptoms is insufficient; we also need to work toward building a life worth living. We may overcome the difficulties of fibromyalgia and discover joy and significance in our daily lives by making the time for self-reflection, pursuing our passions, engaging in meaningful activities, and developing a sense of fulfilment.

Cultivating Mindset for Success

As is well known, fibromyalgia can be a crippling and sometimes overpowering illness that causes weariness, a wide range of symptoms, and pain that prevents a person from living life to the fullest. When faced with such obstacles, it might be simple to slip into a state of pessimism and despair, but it's important to remember that our mindsets have the ability to influence our reality.

Building a resilient mindset starts with positive thinking. We are able to change our attention from what we cannot accomplish to what we can achieve because of this optimistic perspective. Through cognitive restructuring and the substitution of constructive self-talk for negative self-talk, we can start to perceive the potential present in even the most difficult circumstances. Studies have indicated that contemplating positively not only enhances our emotional state but also fortifies our defences against illness and speeds up the recovery process by lowering stress levels.

Another essential component of developing a success-oriented attitude is self-belief. People who have fibromyalgia frequently have self-doubt and persistent doubts about their ability to accomplish their goals. But we can realise our full potential if we have a strong feeling of confidence and self-belief. It is critical that we constantly remind ourselves that having fibromyalgia does not define who we are as people or prevent us from achieving our goals. Despite the obstacles we encounter, we may accomplish excellence in all facets of our lives by identifying and leveraging our abilities.

The third cornerstone of a successful attitude is resilience. It is the capacity to overcome obstacles and see them as chances for personal development. By overcoming setbacks and disappointment, resilience enables us to continue on our path to the best possible health and happiness. According to studies, those who possess high resilience report feeling better about themselves and experiencing less chronic pain. We can weather the fibromyalgia storm by developing resilience, rising stronger from the mist and finding strength in the face of difficulty.

Now that we know how crucial a mindset is to success, let's look at some doable tactics for developing an empowering mindset in relation to managing fibromyalgia. The first step is to start focusing on the things we can control, like our thoughts and behaviours, instead of the things we cannot, like the symptoms of fibromyalgia.

Cognitive reorganisation is a potent method in this respect. This entails recognising and confronting pessimistic ideas and substituting them with realistically optimistic ones. For instance, if we catch ourselves thinking, "My fibromyalgia prevents me from doing the things I used to," we might rephrase this to, "Even with my limitations, there are still many things I can do to lead a fulfilling life." We can progressively change our perspective to one of possibilities and empowerment by deliberately substituting positive thoughts for negative ones.

Self-compassion practise is another useful tactic. Because we might not be able to live up to our own expectations of ourselves, having fibromyalgia can frequently leave us feeling angry and dissatisfied in ourselves. It's crucial to keep in mind nonetheless that our limitations do not define who we are. We can learn to be kind and understanding to ourselves by engaging in self-compassion practises. We can also learn to celebrate our accomplishments, no matter how tiny, and to accept ourselves for who we are. Self-acceptance and self-love are fostered by self-compassion, which enables us to have an optimistic outlook.

Having a network of friends, family, and medical professionals who are sympathetic to our situation and can relate to our experiences is also crucial. Creating a support system of like-minded people who can offer words of encouragement, practical fibromyalgia management advice, and emotional support can go a long way toward enhancing our success mentality. Furthermore, getting expert assistance from coaches or therapists who specialise in chronic illness can offer us helpful direction and resources for developing a success-oriented mindset.

Last but not least, integrating mindfulness exercises into our everyday lives can significantly improve our capacity to develop a resilient attitude. By practising mindfulness, which is being totally present in the moment without passing judgement, we can disengage from unfavourable ideas and feelings and focus our energies on more empowering and positive viewpoints. Deep breathing exercises, body scans, and other mindfulness techniques can help us become more self-aware, manage stress, and create a positive outlook that supports our path to optimum health and well-being.

To sum up, developing a success attitude is an effective strategy for managing fibromyalgia. We can regain our power and lead full, fulfilling lives by adopting a positive outlook, fostering self-belief, and building resilience. The techniques covered in this chapter, including mindfulness training, self-compassion, cognitive restructuring, and creating a support system, can help us on our path to holistic well-being and fibromyalgia mastery. Recall that our mentality serves as both the guide for building a successful, fulfilling life and the solution to managing the symptoms of fibromyalgia.

Embracing Self-Compassion and Acceptance

The emphasis of this subchapter is accepting acceptance and self-compassion as necessary elements of living well with fibromyalgia. It talks about how important it is to take care of oneself, embrace oneself, and recognise one's own accomplishments.

Introduction:

It can be quite difficult to manage fibromyalgia on both a physical and emotional level. It's a chronic illness that frequently causes weariness, pain, and a host of other symptoms that might interfere with day-to-day activities. But it's important to keep in mind that your sickness does not define you. Choosing to accept and be kind to oneself will help you discover happiness and serenity even in the middle of hardships. We will discuss self-acceptance and self-compassion in this chapter and how they can help you have a happy life even with fibromyalgia.

The Power of Self-Compassion:

The act of treating oneself with love, understanding, and empathy is known as self-compassion. It is treating ourselves with the same kindness we would provide to a loved one who is in need. Studies have indicated that the development of self-compassion can have a significant effect on general health and well-being. It can offer consolation and support to fibromyalgia sufferers in the face of ongoing pain and other symptoms.

Our natural tendency is to fight against pain and discomfort when we feel it. But this resistance simply makes things worse for us. We become more aware of our needs and limitations and learn to accept our anguish without passing judgement when we practise self-compassion. This enables us to react to our suffering without becoming frustrated or angry, but rather with kindness and empathy.

Self-care and Self-Acceptance:

In order to control fibromyalgia symptoms and enhance general wellbeing, self-care is essential. It entails making conscious decisions to give your mental and physical well-being first priority. Self-care routines can differ greatly and should be customised to your own requirements and tastes. This can entail changing one's diet, exercising, practising relaxation techniques, changing one's lifestyle, and asking family and friends for assistance.

But self-care is more than just doing physical activities; it also includes accepting who you are. Acknowledging and accepting your present circumstances, including the restrictions and difficulties brought on by fibromyalgia, is the foundation of self-acceptance. It's about learning to accept and value who you are as you are, and letting go of self-criticism and irrational expectations. Focusing on your abilities instead of your limitations is made possible by accepting who you are.

Celebrating Personal Achievements:

Fibromyalgia demands a great deal of fortitude and resiliency to live with. You make decisions and take activities every day to better your well-being and control your symptoms. No matter how minor these accomplishments may appear, they must be celebrated. Acknowledging and appreciating your work might make you feel more accomplished overall and increase your motivation and self-confidence.

Practicing Mindfulness:

A useful technique for developing acceptance and self-compassion is mindfulness. It entails intentionally focusing on the here and now, apart from judgement or attachment. By increasing your awareness of your thoughts, feelings, and physical experiences, mindfulness can help you respond to them with acceptance and compassion.

Consider implementing mindfulness exercises into your everyday schedule. This might be as easy as practising guided meditation or dedicating a short period of time each day to focusing on your breathing. You can develop a greater feeling of acceptance and self-awareness by learning to live in the moment and to be more conscious of your experiences.

Building a Strong Support Network:

Having a solid support system is essential because managing fibromyalgia can be isolating. Be in the company of people who can relate to and comprehend your experiences. Look for physical and online support groups where you can meet people going through similar things. These groups can offer a secure setting for talking about difficulties, exchanging coping mechanisms, and uniting in celebration of accomplishments.

Additionally, think about contacting a therapist or counsellor for expert assistance. They can offer helpful advice and resources to assist you in navigating the psychological aspects of having fibromyalgia. You can cultivate acceptance, self-compassion, and healthy coping methods with the help of therapy.

Conclusion:

Although it's not always simple, learning to accept and love yourself can have a profoundly good effect on many facets of your life. You can survive despite the difficulties posed by fibromyalgia by engaging in self-care, developing self-acceptance, acknowledging your accomplishments, and building a strong support system. Recall that your bravery and fortitude in the face of your disease define you, not your illness itself. Accept self-compassion and the potential that you can have a happy, fulfilled life while having fibromyalgia.

Chapter 11: Future Research and Innovations

Advancements in Fibromyalgia Research

Finding fresh insights into the underlying mechanics of fibromyalgia is one of the most intriguing advances in the field. It has long been believed that fibromyalgia is a central nervous system illness marked by faulty pain processing and extensive pain sensitivity. Although this is still a fair viewpoint, new research has shown how other bodily systems are involved.

For example, new research indicates that immune system malfunction may contribute to the onset of fibromyalgia. Researchers have discovered anomalies in the levels of pro-inflammatory cytokines in fibromyalgia patients, including interleukin-6 (IL-6) and tumour necrosis factor-alpha (TNF-alpha). These results suggest a possible connection between fibromyalgia symptoms and persistent inflammation. It might be feasible to create novel therapies that target the immune system in an effort to reduce pain and other fibromyalgia-related symptoms.

The hunt for putative fibromyalgia biomarkers is another promising field of study. Measurable signs known as biomarkers are useful for tracking the development of a particular ailment or making a diagnosis. Finding trustworthy biomarkers for fibromyalgia would be beneficial not just for early diagnosis but also for tracking therapy efficacy and prognostication.

Numerous biomarkers, including as results from neuroimaging, biochemical markers, and genetic variables, have been the subject of recent investigations. For instance, a number of neuroimaging studies have shown that fibromyalgia patients' brain structure and function differ from those of healthy people. According to one study, those with fibromyalgia exhibited smaller grey matter volumes in several brain areas related to processing pain. These discoveries may aid in the creation of focused therapies and offer insightful information about the neurobiology of fibromyalgia.

Additionally, studies have looked into biochemical markers including substance P and brain-derived neurotrophic factor (BDNF) levels. Increased amounts of substance P, a neuropeptide implicated in the transmission of pain, have been detected in the cerebrospinal fluid of fibromyalgia patients. Conversely, a molecule called BDNF helps nerve cells proliferate and survive. According to studies, BDNF levels are decreased in fibromyalgia patients, which may be related to neuronal malfunction and the emergence of pain sensitization.

Apart from investigating molecular markers, researchers have also focused on the role of genetic variables in the development of fibromyalgia. Certain genetic variants have been found in multiple studies to potentially impact the intensity of symptoms or raise the chance of getting fibromyalgia. For example, a variation in the neurotransmitter metabolism-related COMT gene has been linked to heightened pain sensitivity in fibromyalgia patients. These genetic discoveries open the door to more individualised treatment plans based on a patient's unique genetic makeup in addition to improving our understanding of the illness.

Technological developments have also had a big impact on fibromyalgia diagnosis and therapy. Wearable technology, for instance, can gather information on heart rate variability, activity levels, and sleep patterns. Examples of these devices include smartwatches and fitness trackers. When it comes to keeping an eye on symptoms and figuring out what patterns or triggers can make them worse, this information can be quite helpful. We can enable patients to actively participate in their own care and make educated decisions about their lifestyle and course of treatment by incorporating technology into the management of fibromyalgia.

Virtual reality is another innovative technology that has demonstrated potential in the management of fibromyalgia (VR). By submerging the user in a computer-generated world, virtual reality (VR) stimulates the senses and serves as a pain diversion. Numerous studies have shown how VR can help fibromyalgia patients feel better overall and with less pain. Virtual reality (VR) offers a therapeutic option that is both interesting and non-pharmacological, which has the potential to enhance the quality of life for fibromyalgia sufferers.

To sum up, research on fibromyalgia has advanced our knowledge of the underlying mechanisms of the disorder, possible biomarkers, and the effects of new technology on diagnosis and therapy. These discoveries, which range from figuring out how the immune system functions in fibromyalgia to pinpointing particular genetic variants, could completely alter how this complicated illness is treated. I'm dedicated to giving my patients the best, most individualised care I can by staying on the cutting edge of these developments. By adopting a comprehensive strategy that includes food planning, lifestyle adjustments, counselling, and the incorporation of cutting-edge technologies, we can enable people with fibromyalgia to take charge of their health and fully enjoy life.

Promising Treatment Modalities

Understanding fibromyalgia and the underlying mechanisms that lead to its development has advanced significantly over time. This has opened the door for novel therapeutic approaches that hold great potential for symptom relief and improving general health. We will explore some of these innovative therapies, medicines, and interventions in this chapter. They provide hope and have the potential to completely change the way fibromyalgia is managed.

The creation of novel drugs is among the most fascinating fields of study in the treatment of fibromyalgia. The efficacy and potential negative effects of conventional painkillers, such as opioids and nonsteroidal anti-inflammatory medicines (NSAIDs), are limited. On the other hand, novel therapeutic targets for fibromyalgia have been found recently, which could result in ground-breaking treatments.

Milnacipran, a selective serotonin and norepinephrine reuptake inhibitor (SNRI), is one such drug under investigation. SNRIs have demonstrated potential in the treatment of fibromyalgia symptoms, specifically fatigue and pain. These drugs function by raising serotonin and norepinephrine levels in the brain, which can lessen pain and elevate mood. Preliminary research has demonstrated positive benefits in lowering pain and improving overall quality of life for patients with fibromyalgia, even if the precise mechanism of action is still being investigated.

Innovative approaches are receiving attention in the realm of managing fibromyalgia in addition to pharmaceuticals. With the goal of relieving symptoms and enhancing general health, these treatments try to address the underlying causes of the illness. Transcranial Magnetic Stimulation (TMS), a non-invasive technique that stimulates particular brain regions with magnetic fields, is one such treatment.

TMS has demonstrated potential in lowering fibromyalgia patients' pain and weariness. TMS can assist in blocking pain signals and bringing about relief by focusing on the parts of the brain linked to pain processing. Research have shown that TMS treatment significantly improves quality of life and pain scores. There is still much to learn about the best therapy approaches and long-term effects of TMS, but it has enormous promise as a non-pharmacological intervention for fibromyalgia.

Another effective therapeutic option for fibromyalgia is cognitive-behavioral therapy (CBT). The goal of this therapy is to change unfavourable beliefs and actions that fuel pain perception. CBT can enable people to better control their symptoms and enhance their general quality of life by assisting them in creating coping mechanisms and strengthening their self-management abilities.

Studies have demonstrated that CBT can help fibromyalgia sufferers sleep better, feel less pain, and have better psychological health. Cognitive Behavioral Therapy (CBT) offers a holistic approach to managing fibromyalgia by treating the psychological and emotional aspects of the disorder. It gives people the resources they need to deal with the difficulties of having the illness, which eventually results in a more contented and pleasurable existence.

Complementary and alternative medicine (CAM) approaches are a promising new therapeutic option for fibromyalgia. CAM includes many different types of treatments, such as herbal remedies, yoga, meditation, and acupuncture. These methods concentrate on using the body's inherent healing capacity to reduce symptoms and enhance general health.

For instance, acupuncture has demonstrated potential in lowering pain and enhancing the quality of sleep for those with fibromyalgia. Acupuncture helps produce endorphins, serotonin, and other neurotransmitters that can help regulate pain perception by stimulating certain spots on the body. On the flip side, yoga and meditation encourage rest, lower stress levels, and enhance general physical and mental wellbeing.

Herbal therapies with possible anti-inflammatory and pain-relieving effects, such turmeric and St. John's wort, have also drawn interest. Although further investigation is required to determine the ideal dosages and compositions of these treatments, they present a safe and natural substitute for conventional pharmaceuticals.

A comprehensive fibromyalgia management plan that incorporates these alternative strategies might offer people a range of solutions to meet their specific requirements and preferences. Through the integration of pharmaceutical, therapeutic, and intervention benefits, patients can maximise treatment results and see a notable improvement in their overall quality of life and symptoms.

In conclusion, there are potential new therapy options for fibromyalgia that are constantly being developed in this field. For those suffering from fibromyalgia, there is hope thanks to new drugs that target particular neurochemical imbalances as well as creative therapies and interventions that target the underlying processes of the disorder. Through the adoption of a comprehensive and holistic approach to care, people can acquire the necessary tools to manage their symptoms and live a life that is full of energy and wellness.As a medical doctor and health and wellness coach, I am committed to staying up-to-date with the latest research and advancements in fibromyalgia treatment to offer my patients the most effective and comprehensive management strategies. Together, we can navigate the complexities of fibromyalgia and empower individuals to live their best lives.

Integrative Approaches to Fibromyalgia

The complicated illness known as fibromyalgia is typified by persistent pain, exhaustion, irregular sleep patterns, and cognitive problems. The main focus of traditional Western medicine is frequently on using drugs like antidepressants and painkillers to control symptoms. Although some people may find success with these treatments, they frequently are unable to address the underlying causes and offer complete relief. Herein lies the role of integrative medicine.

Integrative medicine places a strong emphasis on treating the patient as a whole, mind, body, and spirit. It acknowledges that achieving health and wellbeing calls for a customised, comprehensive strategy rather than a one-size-fits-all one. We are able to offer a more thorough and successful fibromyalgia treatment plan by fusing the finest aspects of complementary medicine with traditional medication.

Reducing the need for medication is one of the main advantages of integrative medicine. Medication can be helpful in managing symptoms, but it can also have a number of negative effects and not always treat the underlying cause of the pain or discomfort. Complementary therapies can help us repair the body naturally and lessen the need for prescription drugs by combining practises like acupuncture, yoga, and massage therapy.

According to research, fibromyalgia sufferers may benefit especially from acupuncture, an ancient Chinese medicine procedure that involves inserting tiny needles into specified body locations. Acupuncture has been shown in studies to help with pain management, better sleep, and overall life quality enhancement. We can encourage balance in the energy pathways and activate the body's natural healing powers by applying pressure to particular acupuncture points.

Yoga is another effective technique in the integrative toolbox. Yoga, which emphasises deep breathing, moderate movement, and mindfulness, has several advantages for those with fibromyalgia. Yoga has been demonstrated to enhance general physical and mental well-being, lessen pain and stiffness, and enhance the quality of sleep. Yoga also promotes self-awareness and self-compassion, two qualities that are critical for handling the psychological and emotional elements of fibromyalgia.

Another complementary therapy that might give fibromyalgia sufferers much-needed respite is massage therapy. This manual method can ease pain, promote better circulation, and release tense muscles. People with fibromyalgia can benefit physically and psychologically by engaging with a trained massage therapist, including reduced anxiety and enhanced pain perception.

The management of fibromyalgia necessitates lifestyle improvements in addition to complementary therapy. These adjustments cover a wide range of day-to-day activities, such as stress reduction, diet, and physical activity. People can minimise the effects of fibromyalgia symptoms and maximise their general well-being by leading a balanced and healthy lifestyle.

Even though it can be difficult at first, exercise is crucial for those with fibromyalgia. Frequent exercise has been demonstrated to lessen pain, enhance mood, enhance sleep quality, and improve general physical fitness. Exercise should be done carefully though, as using too much energy can make symptoms worse. The secret is to strike a balance between rest and mild, low-impact exercises like walking or swimming.

Another important factor in the management of fibromyalgia is nutrition. Studies have demonstrated that some foods, like those rich in antioxidants and anti-inflammatory qualities, can aid in lowering inflammation and symptom relief. Conversely, refined sweets, processed meals, and caffeine could exacerbate discomfort and exhaustion. Consulting with a licenced dietitian can help you develop a customised eating plan that promotes your best health and wellbeing.

Another essential component of managing fibromyalgia is stress management. It has been demonstrated that stress increases symptom severity and adds to the condition's overall burden. Relaxation techniques, deep breathing, and meditation are examples of mind-body practises that can assist in lowering stress and fostering calm. Furthermore, it can be quite useful for general wellbeing to partake in joyful and relaxing activities, including being creative or spending time in nature.

People with fibromyalgia must incorporate a range of self-care approaches and coping skills. These methods can aid in symptom management, raise general wellbeing, and improve quality of life. There are a lot of resources and methods to investigate, ranging from biofeedback and cognitive-behavioral therapy to heat therapy and hydrotherapy. It's critical to collaborate closely with a healthcare provider who can help you choose the methods that will best meet your unique requirements.

To sum up, integrative methods of managing fibromyalgia provide a detailed and customised road map for people looking for relief from this complicated illness. The integration of complementary therapies, lifestyle adjustments, and mind-body practises with conventional medication can effectively target the underlying causes of fibromyalgia and bolster the body's inherent healing capabilities. I have faith that by using this all-encompassing strategy, we can enable people to take back control of their health and prosper in spite of the difficulties posed by fibromyalgia.

Patient Perspectives and Future Directions

Patient advocacy is essential for debunking misconceptions about fibromyalgia and removing obstacles to getting the right care. I have a limited amount of power as a medical expert to inform people about this illness and provide them with the assistance they require. The patients are the ones who really know what struggles they endure on a daily basis, and it is through their advocacy work that significant change may be enacted.

Participating actively in research projects is one way that individuals may advocate for themselves and other fibromyalgia sufferers. Research studies and clinical trials are essential for expanding our knowledge of this complicated illness and creating fresh approaches to therapy. Patients who take part in these studies not only add to the corpus of information about fibromyalgia but also get access to novel treatments and therapies that might not be found in other places.

A greater understanding of the significance of incorporating patient viewpoints in the research process has emerged in recent years. Patients are becoming more and more involved in the planning, carrying out, and interpreting of research because researchers recognise that their special perspectives and experiences can illuminate topics that may have gone unnoticed in more conventional research methods. This cooperative strategy has the power to completely transform the industry and produce solutions that are genuinely patient-centered.

The creation of patient-reported outcome measures is an excellent illustration of how patients can participate in research (PROMs). With the use of these instruments, patients can self-report their functioning, quality of life, and symptoms, giving a more complete and accurate picture of how fibromyalgia affects their day-to-day activities. PROMs have shown to be quite helpful in determining the actual cost of the illness and evaluating the efficacy of various treatments. We can guarantee that the measurements encompass the entire spectrum of experiences and results that hold significance for patients by integrating patient viewpoints into these outcome assessments.

In addition, involving patients in research empowers people and offers them a sense of control over their illness in addition to improving the findings' relevance and applicability. It encourages collaboration amongst patients, researchers, and medical personnel, resulting in a collaborative atmosphere that propels advancement and innovation.

It is crucial to stress the significance of cooperative efforts in influencing the direction of fibromyalgia research and management, in addition to patient advocacy and research engagement. In order to communicate ideas, share expertise, and work toward shared objectives, healthcare professionals, researchers, patients, and advocacy groups must collaborate. This multidisciplinary approach facilitates the creation of integrative and holistic treatment solutions as well as a thorough understanding of the problem.

We can investigate promising paths including complementary and alternative therapies, psychological interventions, and self-help methods by working together. A complicated illness that affects people physically, psychologically, and emotionally is fibromyalgia. Therefore, complete management requires a multimodal and multidimensional strategy. We can include a variety of strategies that cater to the different needs of individuals with fibromyalgia by utilising the knowledge of professionals from other professions.

To sum up, patient viewpoints are extremely helpful in the field of managing and researching fibromyalgia. To spur innovation and advancement, patient advocacy, research engagement, and teamwork are crucial. We can make sure that the solutions we design are truly patient-centered and customised to meet their specific needs by involving patients at every stage of the process. The lives of those who suffer with fibromyalgia can be significantly improved by us working together and being united.

Chapter 12: Resources and Support

Online Resources and Websites

1. National Fibromyalgia Association (NFA):

The NFA is a respectable organisation that works to raise awareness of fibromyalgia and offer assistance to those who have it. Their website is a veritable gold mine of information, with articles, research updates, and helpful symptom management advice. In addition, they provide a community forum where you may interact with people who share your experiences. The NFA also often organises webinars and educational programmes that might help you learn more about managing fibromyalgia.

2. Fibromyalgia Action UK:

The website of Fibromyalgia Action UK is a great resource for people in the United Kingdom. They offer self-management strategies, evidence-based knowledge, and helpful guidance to assist you in overcoming the difficulties of having fibromyalgia. Additionally, you can connect with other people going through similar challenges by using the database of local support groups available on their website. Additionally, you can call their helpline to ask problems and get advice from their team of experienced volunteers.

3. Mayo Clinic Fibromyalgia Page:

The Mayo Clinic is renowned for its superiority in patient care and medical research. They provide a plethora of information on symptoms, causes, diagnosis, and treatment choices on their extensive fibromyalgia website. You can learn more about your disease by utilising the interactive tools, videos, and in-depth publications available. In addition, the Mayo Clinic offers guidance for loved ones and caregivers, stressing the value of having a strong support system when attempting to manage fibromyalgia.

4. Cochrane Library:

For reliable sources of systematic reviews and meta-analyses on a range of medical issues, including fibromyalgia, consult the Cochrane

Library. These reviews offer evidence-based management and treatment recommendations by summarising and analysing the available research. You can find high-quality research papers that can help you make decisions about your healthcare by going to their website and searching for topics relevant to fibromyalgia.

5. Fibromyalgia Network:

The Fibromyalgia Network was founded in 1988 and has provided fibromyalgia sufferers with trustworthy information for more than thirty years. Numerous resources, such as articles, bulletins, and even online courses on topics like pain management, exercise, and mental health, are available on their website. Additionally, they have a bookstore stocked with suggested books and DVDs covering a range of topics related to managing fibromyalgia.

6. The Mighty:

An online group called The Mighty is dedicated to empowering and helping people who suffer from long-term conditions like fibromyalgia. On their website, individuals who have lived with fibromyalgia for a long time share their personal narratives, articles, and tips. It's a great way to meet people who understand your difficulties, get support and motivation, and learn about various coping mechanisms.

7. Chronic Pain Partners:

A non-profit group called Chronic Pain Partners offers assistance and services to those with long-term pain disorders, such as fibromyalgia. They have educational resources, webinars, and online support groups available on their website to help you manage your symptoms and enhance your quality of life. They also include a network of medical professionals who focus on managing chronic pain, which enables you to locate professionals that genuinely comprehend your requirements.

8. FibroCenter:

An online resource called FibroCenter was created especially to meet the needs of people who have fibromyalgia. On their website, you can find practical resources, self-help methods, and evidence-based information for managing the symptoms of fibromyalgia. They provide a variety of online workshops and courses on subjects like nutrition, stress relief, pain treatment, and good sleep hygiene. You can get the knowledge and resources you need to take charge of your fibromyalgia experience with FibroCenter.

9. FibroTrack:

With the cutting-edge web application FibroTrack, you may monitor your drug intake, mood, energy levels, and symptoms. By keeping an eye on these areas of your life, you can identify trends and stressors that might make your fibromyalgia symptoms worse. In-depth data that you can share with your healthcare practitioner through FibroTrack also help you communicate with them more effectively and create individualised treatment strategies.

10. Your Health e-Clinic:

An online resource called Your Health e-Clinic provides individualised health coaching and assistance to those with fibromyalgia and other chronic pain problems. Their team of specialists may offer advice on coping mechanisms, nutrition planning, stress reduction methods, and lifestyle adjustments. Working with a health coach can improve your general well-being by providing you with individualised, all-encompassing support that is catered to your particular needs.

In conclusion, people with fibromyalgia can find a plethora of information, support, and useful advice on the websites and online resources included in this subchapter. These trustworthy resources can act as your guide for comprehensive fibromyalgia care, whether you're seeking for instructional materials, research updates, or self-help strategies. Don't forget to take your time exploring these resources and choose the ones that best suit your needs and objectives. By working together, we can overcome the obstacles associated with having fibromyalgia and enable ourselves to have happy, full lives.

Support Organizations and Helplines

As a physician and health and wellness coach, I am aware of the difficulties that fibromyalgia sufferers deal with on a daily basis. It can be quite difficult to manage the symptoms of this chronic illness, therefore it's critical to have a solid support network. I'm committed to giving you the tools you need to manage your fibromyalgia because of this.

We will look at the support groups and hotlines created especially for fibromyalgia sufferers in this chapter. These organisations provide a wide range of services, including financial aid, emotional support, and advice on healthcare. Let's get started and investigate the useful tools at your disposal.

Emotional Support:

Fibromyalgia can make emotional life difficult. Feelings of loneliness and despair are frequently brought on by the pain, exhaustion, and other symptoms. Having a solid support network is essential to preserving mental health. Thankfully, fibromyalgia sufferers can find emotional support from a number of groups.

The Fibromyalgia Support Alliance is one such group. They provide virtual forums for people with fibromyalgia to interact with one another. These support groups offer a secure environment where you can talk about your experiences, get answers to your questions, and learn insightful things from others who genuinely get what you're going through.

The National Fibromyalgia Association is another excellent source of information. They provide a skilled volunteer-run helpline with emotional assistance and guidance. The helpline is here to help, whether you just need someone to chat to or have concerns about dealing with your symptoms.

Financial Assistance:

The cost of treating fibromyalgia can be high. The financial hardship can exacerbate an already difficult condition with more medical bills, drug expenditures, and possibly fewer work hours. Nonetheless, those with fibromyalgia who require financial support can turn to certain organisations.

Grants are available from the Fibromyalgia Foundation to qualified persons to assist with the expenses of managing fibromyalgia. These awards can be applied to a range of costs, including prescription drugs, therapy sessions, and medical expenditures. The foundation is committed to assisting as many people as possible, and applying for a grant is a simple process.

Healthcare Guidance:

Handling a complicated ailment like fibromyalgia can make navigating the healthcare system difficult and intimidating. That is the role of associations such as the American Chronic Pain Association. They offer tools and advice for locating the best medical professionals, comprehending available treatments, and sticking up for yourself as a fibromyalgia sufferer.

Furthermore, the Fibromyalgia Research and Treatment Center provides thorough medical advice designed especially for individuals with fibromyalgia. They have a group of professionals who can offer tailored guidance and recommendations because they comprehend the particular difficulties in managing this illness. The centre is here to support you whether you want to look into alternative treatment options or need assistance contacting a fibromyalgia specialist.

Apart from the aforementioned organisations, there are multiple helplines that offer specific assistance and support related to fibromyalgia. One such resource is the National Fibromyalgia Community Helpline. They give a toll-free number where you can get in touch with knowledgeable volunteers who can offer assistance, resources, and information. The helpline is open from Monday to Friday, so you can call it anytime you need advice or assistance.

I strongly advise you to utilise these excellent resources. Building a network of support and taking advantage of the resources at your disposal can have a big impact on how you manage your fibromyalgia. Recall that you are not alone on this path.

To sum up, this subsection has furnished details regarding the diverse support groups and hotlines accessible for individuals suffering with fibromyalgia. These options, which range from financial aid to emotional support to medical advice, might help you deal with the difficulties of having fibromyalgia. I urge you to get in touch with us and make use of these helpful resources. Never forget that you deserve all of the help and support you can get as you work to improve your fibromyalgia management.

Community Forums and Support Groups

As a physician and health and wellness coach, I have personally seen the transforming potential of fibromyalgia patients' community forums and support groups. These sites offer a secure and welcoming environment where people can connect with others going through comparable struggles. Patients gain comfort, understanding, and a steadfast source of support from these relationships.

The opportunity to connect with people who can really relate to your experiences is what sets community forums and support groups apart. There are many people in these forums who have experienced the same things as you, including the incapacitating symptoms, frustrations, and difficulties dealing with the intricacies of fibromyalgia. It's a journey together that strengthens bonds of friendship and support.

Joining a community forum or support group offers the chance to share knowledge, tactics, and coping processes, which is one of the main advantages. Participants can share and learn from each other's experiences in an open and honest manner here. These little pearls of wisdom, whether they are about how to manage discomfort or how to save energy, can be quite helpful.

Additionally, community forums and support groups serve as a channel for the most recent findings and available treatments. Members frequently discuss innovations in medicine, achievements in science, and complementary medicines that have helped them. This abundance of knowledge guarantees that you are not alone in your search for useful fibromyalgia management techniques.

Let's investigate a few of the online resources designed especially for the fibromyalgia community. Discussion forums are available on websites like "Fibromyalgia Network," "National Fibromyalgia Association," and "Fibromyalgia Action UK," where people may interact, exchange ideas, and feel a feeling of community. These platforms are extremely beneficial since they make it easy to interact with people whenever it's convenient for you, right from the comfort of your own home.

Several fibromyalgia support groups have emerged on social media platforms in addition to these online forums. There are numerous fibromyalgia-focused Facebook groups where people may share their experiences, give advice, and support one another. Real-time communication is possible in these communities, and you can build a network of people who will support you in times of need.

The benefits of digital environments notwithstanding, in-person communication still has tremendous force. Attending in-person support groups offers people a special chance to form deep connections with people in their community. Having a solid support network can be especially helpful at trying times when being there physically can make a huge difference.

You can get in touch with groups like the American Chronic Pain Association, neighbourhood community centres, or even your own physician to locate in-person support groups. These groups frequently come together to exchange stories, talk about coping mechanisms, and even partake in activities that enhance general wellbeing. It may be incredibly empowering and inspiring to be with people who genuinely understand your experience.

It's crucial to remember that, despite their many advantages, community forums and support groups cannot replace expert medical advice. They can, however, be a useful addition to your therapy regimen, enhancing your understanding and offering emotional support.

In conclusion, fibromyalgia sufferers really benefit from participating in community forums and support groups. They provide a forum for people to interact, exchange stories, and find comfort in one another's understanding. These networks offer a vital source of knowledge, direction, and unconditional support, regardless of whether you choose to join in-person support groups or participate in online discussions. Recall that you are not travelling alone, and that by working together, we can overcome the difficulties caused by fibromyalgia.

Additional Reading and Recommended Books

Memoirs have a special ability to vividly depict the human experience, enabling us to empathise with the hardships and victories of others. Regarding fibromyalgia, they offer an insight into the lives of individuals coping with this persistent ailment. Sarah Cashfeld's "The Diary of a Fibromyalgia Warrior" is one such memoir that I heartily suggest. Sarah describes her experience with fibromyalgia in this moving and emotional narrative, from the first signs of the condition to discovering her way to mental and physical recovery. Anyone who has ever personally dealt with the difficulties of fibromyalgia will be able to relate to her honest and unvarnished stories.

"Invisible: How Young Women with Serious Health Issues Navigate Work, Relationships, and the Pressure to Seem Just Fine" by Michele Lent Hirsch is another memoir that is well worth reading. This anthology includes narratives from several young women who are coping with chronic health conditions, such as fibromyalgia, but it is not exclusively focused on the condition. Through their personal accounts, Hirsch illuminates the particular challenges that contemporary young women experience and offers insightful information about the difficulties associated with managing chronic illness while attempting to lead regular lives in all spheres of life.

Going on to self-help books, "Fibromyalgia Freedom" by Kathleen Stengel is a great choice. Stengel provides a thorough guide to comprehending fibromyalgia and creating a toolkit of techniques for efficiently managing its symptoms, drawing on her personal experience with the illness. This book offers a comprehensive approach to managing fibromyalgia, ranging from helpful suggestions on diet and exercise to methods for lowering stress and improving sleep. Anyone looking to take charge of their fibromyalgia symptoms will find this guide to be a great resource due to Stengel's deep knowledge and compassionate tone.

I suggest Dr. Ginevra Liptan's "The FibroManual: A Complete Fibromyalgia Treatment Guide for You and Your Doctor" for anyone interested in learning more about the scientific components of fibromyalgia. As a physician with a focus on fibromyalgia, Dr. Liptan offers a thorough approach to diagnosing and managing the condition by fusing her experience with the most recent research findings. This book provides evidence-based treatment techniques and an explanation of the science underlying fibromyalgia, enabling patients and healthcare professionals to manage fibromyalgia effectively.

Additionally, I recommend Dr. Jackie Gardner-"The Nix's Mindfulness Solution to Pain: Step-by-Step Techniques for Chronic Pain Management" for a more thorough knowledge of the mind-body link and its function in fibromyalgia. This book examines how to effectively manage chronic pain, including fibromyalgia, with mindfulness and meditation practises. Dr. Gardner-Nix provides helpful advice on how to use mindfulness-based techniques to your everyday life so that you can become more resilient and self-aware when dealing with pain.

Dr. Melissa Congdon's book "The Everything Guide to Fibromyalgia: An Integrated Approach to Managing Pain and Wellness" offers a thorough summary of all the therapy choices available if you're interested in investigating complementary and alternative therapies for fibromyalgia. This book discusses a variety of complementary therapies, including yoga, herbal remedies, and massage therapy, and assesses how well they work for treating fibromyalgia symptoms. By providing readers with evidence-based knowledge and helpful guidance, Dr. Congdon enables them to make well-informed decisions on their course of treatment.

If you want to learn more about fibromyalgia, these suggested books are only the beginning. Keep in mind that every person's experience with this illness is different, so it's critical to consider a variety of viewpoints and strategies. These books will offer additional insights and support on your fibromyalgia journey, regardless of whether you are looking for solace in memoirs, useful advice in self-help books, or a deeper understanding through scientific literature.

To sum up, more reading about fibromyalgia might be a great way to supplement the information and techniques included in this book. Through exploring these many viewpoints and evidence-based insights, you can learn more about this intricate illness and uncover fresh approaches to effectively manage your fibromyalgia.

Milton Keynes UK
Ingram Content Group UK Ltd.
UKHW011314120324
439381UK00009B/556